Drug-Induced Oral Complications

Sarah Cousty · Sara Laurencin-Dalicieux

Editors

Drug-Induced Oral Complications

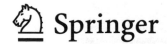

Editors
Sarah Cousty
Oral Surgery Oral Medecine
Department, Dental Faculty
Paul Sabatier University
Toulouse
France

Sara Laurencin-Dalicieux
Periodontology Department, Dental
Faculty
Paul Sabatier University
Toulouse
France

Oral Surgery Oral Medecine Department
CHU de Toulouse
Toulouse
France

Periodontology Department
CHU de Toulouse
Toulouse
France

LAPLACE, UMR CNRS 5213
Paul Sabatier University
Toulouse
France

CERPOP, UMR INSERM 1295
Paul Sabatier University
Toulouse
France

ISBN 978-3-030-66975-1   ISBN 978-3-030-66973-7   (eBook)
https://doi.org/10.1007/978-3-030-66973-7

This Springer imprint is published by the registered company Springer Nature Switzerland AG
The registered company address is: Gewerbestrasse 11, 6330 Cham, Switzerland

General Introduction

Medications are part of our patient's daily lives: antibiotics, analgesics, antiarrhythmics, antidepressants, anticoagulants, hypoglycemics, immunosuppressors, immunomodulators, and others. In addition to their expected and necessary therapeutic effects, drugs can induce complications or side effects, many of which can be involved in oral complications with variable localization, severity, and frequency, such as ulcerations, lichenoid reactions, pigmentation, and bullous reactions.

Some drugs present a direct toxicity, particularly on bone tissue, such as bisphosphonates or denosumab that prevent bone mass loss (osteoporosis and bone metastasis). Others (such as antithrombotic therapies) can increase hemorrhagic risks and cause spontaneous bleeding or surgical complications or can enhance infectious risks such as chemotherapy and biotherapy.

All of them have an impact on the patient's well-being and quality of life ranging from a slight discomfort to a life-threatening emergency and unfortunately are often under and misdiagnosed.

This book is intended for doctors, dentists, nurses, and specialists or not of the oral cavity. The aim is to help clinicians in diagnosing these adverse effects, according to the elementary lesion, by pointing out the most important oral complications related to drugs in terms of prevalence and side effects, particularly in relation to recently developed therapies.

We would like to thank our colleagues (clinicians, surgeons, drug safety specialists) for their contribution to this collaborative work.

Contents

Adverse Drug Reactions, Iatrogenic Diseases, Drug Safety, and Pharmacovigilance: Importance and Interest for Patients and Their Physicians

Jean-Louis Montastruc, Haleh Bagheri,
Genevieve Durrieu, Isabelle Lacroix,
and François Montastruc

1 Introduction

Recent withdrawals of drugs for safety reasons (cerivastatin, rofecoxib, rimonabant, sibutramine, nimesulide, benfluorex, or rosiglitazone

J.-L. Montastruc (✉)
French National Academy of Medicine ("Académie Nationale de Médecine"), Medical Pharmacology, Faculty of Medicine, University of Toulouse, Toulouse, France

Department of Medical and Clinical Pharmacology, Toulouse PharmacoVigilance and PharmacoEpidemiology Center, Toulouse University Hospital, Toulouse, France
e-mail: jean-louis.montastruc@univ-tlse3.fr

H. Bagheri · G. Durrieu · I. Lacroix
Department of Medical and Clinical Pharmacology, Toulouse PharmacoVigilance and PharmacoEpidemiology Center, Toulouse University Hospital, Toulouse, France
e-mail: bagheri.h@chu-toulouse.fr; genevieve. durrieu@univ-tlse3.fr; isabelle.lacroix@univ-tlse3.fr

F. Montastruc
Faculty of Medicine, Department of Medical and Clinical Pharmacology, University of Toulouse, Toulouse, France

Toulouse PharmacoVigilance and PharmacoEpidemiology Center, Toulouse University Hospital, Toulouse, France
e-mail: montastruc.f2@chu-toulouse.fr

...) have focused interest of health professionals on pharmacovigilance (PV). These "affairs" underline the difficulties of monitoring drug use and drug safety in daily practice. This review describes the clinical importance of drug safety, PV, and iatrogenic diseases.

2 Definition and Organization of Pharmacovigilance

Developed around the world since the 1960s as a result of the thalidomide scandal, and in France, from the mid-1970s after the observation of bismuth encephalopathies, the aim of PV is the study of ADRs (adverse drugs reactions) defined as "harmful and unwanted reactions to a drug occurring at normal dosages or after misuse." According to the law of 29 December 2011, the purpose of pharmacovigilance is to monitor, evaluate, prevent, and manage the risk of adverse effects resulting from the use of drugs. The notion of PV is, of course, reminiscent of the etymological double meaning of the Greek "*pharmakon,*" both remedy and poison.

ADRs are frequent: they correspond to 5–10% of hospitalizations, 5–10% of outpatients' consultations, and occur in 25–30% of patients hospitalized. In France, a study from the Regional

Pharmacovigilance Centers (CRPV) found that 140,000 admissions to hospitals (psychiatric hospitals excluded) per year are related to an ADR. This number is higher than that of myocardial infarction occurring each year in France and corresponds to a higher cost than the annual management of diabetes. From these data, it can be estimated that 10–30,000 deaths are, each year in France, related to an ADR. These ADRs concern both prescription drugs and self-medication drugs, including the so-called advisory products, consumer medications. These ADRs can take any clinical picture (not only cutaneous, cardiac, neurological, psychiatric but also fractures, falls). Moreover, they could be prevented in about 30–50% of cases. The prevention of these avoidable effects, and especially those explained by the pharmacodynamic properties of drugs, must make it possible to optimize the proper use of the drug. Finally, ADRs are the fourth leading cause of death in industrialized countries.

Thus, ADRs are too frequent. How to limit them? It seems impossible to completely eliminate them, because we cannot predict and control the susceptibility and therefore the reactions of each patient receiving a drug. There are several explications, the first being the extraordinary genetic diversity of humans, which does not predict the responsiveness of all individuals to drugs, but only the largest number. We can only recall emergence of susceptibility genes, associated diseases, and interactions with xenobiotics, like other drugs, food, and environmental contaminants. This underlines the importance of pharmacogenetics and pharmacogenomics approaches in PV, in order to prevent occurrence of ADRs in some at-risk patients.

The objectives of PV are multiple: detection of ADRs (signal evaluation), quantification of risk (prevalence, incidence of ADRs), comparison of risk within the same pharmacological or therapeutic class, primary and secondary prevention of drug risk, information of health professionals and public, and finally better pharmacological knowledge of drugs for their proper use. PV also allows the identification of new therapeutic indications, from the discovery of an ADR of already marketed drugs. The clas-

sic examples are the antihypertensive action of beta-blockers and the hypoglycemic effect of sulfonamides prescribed in infections. Finally, the most recent missions of pharmacovigilance relate to the management of the health risk, both at national level (in collaboration with the National Drug Agencies) and at a regional level (in close partnership with the Regional Health Agencies).

In France, pharmacovigilance is organized on a decentralized basis from the network of 31 *Regional Centers of PV (RCPV)* working in collection, validation, and evaluation of ADRs. RCPV are also in charge of drug information to health professionals and now to patients. CRPVs are also involved in training on proper drug use, as well as, at the request of the French Drug Agency (ANSM), surveys, and expertise on safety of medicines. They also carry out research on drug safety, a neglected topic in medical research.

In addition to this public PV system, pharmaceutical companies must also monitor drug safety for their medicines. ADRs that they collect in a country are transmitted to the national authorities, in France (ANSM), European (European Medicine Agency EMA), and international (World Health Organization WHO), and thus are available for any investigation of PV, in case of alert. Firms also must mandatorily send periodic safety reports on their products to health authorities.

Finally, in Europe, regulatory decisions are in charge of the European Pharmacovigilance Risk Assessment Committee (PRAC) which takes all decisions to improve drug safety, information, restriction of use or withdrawals.

3   Methods in Pharmacovigilance

Methods for quantifying the risk of drug use are numerous, ranging from experimental pharmacology and toxicology observations to the results of clinical trials and pharmacoepidemiology data. It should be made clear that, contrary to the study of the clinical efficacy of drugs, the notion of "level of evidence" is not suitable for the evaluation of drug risk. In PV, signal comes most often from multiple sources: preclinical pharmacology, clinical trials, spontaneous reports, or pharmacoepidemiological analyses. Some methods are more appropriate, but none should be neglected. Thus, decision-making in PV remains difficult, since it requires taking into account all the basic, clinical, and epidemiological data on diseases and drugs.

The data obtained during the preclinical development of the drug (fundamental pharmacology and toxicology), allowing to understand the mechanism of favorable as well as noxious actions of drugs, can already represent one of evidence in PV. For example, it has recently been demonstrated that the affinity of pioglitazone for PPAR receptors (α as well as γ), known since the first stages of the development of these hypoglycemic drugs, made it possible to explain, as well as to predict, the occurrence of bladder cancer, a risk identified much later in the life of this drug.

Clinical trials, because they correspond to the first use of the drug in humans, are one of the sources of information on ADRs. However, they are better suited to the study of benefit than risk of drugs. Their limits for the evaluation of adverse effects are summed up by the "five too" formula: (1) they are too brief, (2) their indications are too narrow, (3) they involve a too limited age group (including too few children and/or older people), (4) the number of patients participating is too small, and (5) they include too simple medical situations. For example, pregnant women do not usually participate in testing new drugs. To this list, we can add the current trend of early drug approval AMM, which also reduces premarket evaluation. However, despite their limitations, clinical trials can sometimes give important information, as in 2004 for the withdrawal of rofecoxib, following the detection of an increased thrombotic risk in the APPROVe clinical trial.

Thus, the true follow-up of ADRs is performed in phase IV (i.e., after drug marketing). The basic method in pharmacovigilance is then represented by *spontaneous reporting*, i.e., reports by health professionals of ADRs to their Regional Pharmacovigilance Centers. Since 2011, the new European law made mandatory to report not only "serious" or "unexpected" ADRs but now "any suspected ADR." This statement concerns doctors, dentists, midwives, and pharmacists. It is also "possible" to report for other health professionals as well as, since 2011, for patients and patient associations. This last point (notifications by patients) is a new added value for pharmacovigilance and drug safety.

Spontaneous reporting has several strengths: it is simple, inexpensive, involves all drugs throughout their whole life, can generate a signal, formulate a hypothesis, and describe the common characteristics from the case series. This spontaneous reporting often suffers from a low informativeness of the reports as well as the underreporting, which does not allow to really know the real incidence of the ADR in population. The causes of underreporting are well identified: ignorance of reporting requirements, insufficient training of health professionals in PV and reporting requirements, lack of motivation of health professionals, fear of appearing insufficiently trained and informed, fears of prosecution, and lack of return from health authorities. In addition, the spontaneous reporting does not allow knowing the true frequency (incidence or prevalence) of ADRs. However, it remains the basic method in PV, because, unlike clinical trials, which only reveal "very frequent" (that is to say, a frequency greater than 1 in 10) or "frequent" (between 1/10 and 1/100) adverse events, spontaneous reporting is the only method today allowing the surveillance of any type of ADR, whatever its frequency, and in particular the "very rare" ones (defined as less than 1 per 10,000).

Reports of ADRs are then documented and analyzed from a medical and pharmacological point of view in order to evaluate the *causality assessment (also called imputability")*, i.e., the relationship between drug(s) and ADR occurrence. Causality assessment's score includes two components: first, the so-called "extrinsic" accountability, i.e., bibliography ("B"), i.e., data present (or not) in reference books in clinical pharmacology and pharmacovigilance, the summary of product characteristics (SPC), or literature; second, "intrinsic" accountability, a combination of the "chronological" score and the "semiological" score. The chronological score (*C*) is established from three data: (1) time of ADR onset after drug intake ("challenge"); (2) evolution of the clinical picture, especially after withdrawal of the suspected drug ("dechallenge"); and (3) drug "rechallenge" (when possible, of course) with or without ADR reappearance. The semiological score (*S*) is constructed from clinical and/or paraclinical data found in the clinical observation and obviously takes into account the exclusion or not of other diagnoses (differential diagnoses). Finally, combination of these two scores, *C* plus *S*, defines the intrinsic imputability score, called "*I*", ranging from *I*0 ("excluded") to *I*4 ("very likely"). Once imputed, the pharmacovigilance report does not remain in dusty drawers but is transmitted to the national drug agency to be registered, first in the national pharmacovigilance database and then in the WHO pharmacovigilance database at Uppsala VigiBase®. Thus, as soon as a question on safety of one or more drugs will arise, PV specialists in PV centers and health authorities will be able to see if other cases were already published in order to establish an alert and to discuss the new benefit/harm of the drug(s).

Pharmacovigilance centers do not only have a role in signal detection. They are also independent sources of ***drug information*** to which all practitioners should refer to obtain up-to-date information on ADRs, drug effectiveness, drug interactions, or use in at-risk populations (elderly, renal insufficiency, hepatic insufficiency, pregnant, or lactating women...). This notion of information from PV centers is now crucial for prescribers. Thus, the pharmacovigilance center must now be considered as a clinical and medical-pharmaceutical unit performing:

1. ADRs diagnosis and management.
2. Independent information on drugs.
3. Optimization of drug prescription in general and in at-risk subjects.

Spontaneous reports thus allow detecting signals. Later, ***pharmacoepidemiology*** quantifies the drug risk through additional studies applying the methods of epidemiology to the study and quantification of ADRs.

Thus, pharmacoepidemiological methods extend to a populational level the data of spontaneous reporting. It could be first descriptive cross-sectional studies, such as "one day" or intensive pharmacovigilance follow-up, as for influenza A (H1N1) vaccines during the winter of 2009–2010. However, these methods do not allow the evaluation of "very rare" ADRs (<1 per 10,000). Cohort studies have also an important place in PV. They have the advantage of being prospective, allowing the calculation of Relative Risk (RR). They allow to eliminate some biases such as memory ones. However, they require a large number of patients, are time-consuming and costly, are inadequate for rare ADRs, and cannot overcome other biases (such as selection, classification, confusion, or loss of subjects). They are useful for ADRs with an incidence greater than 1 per 1000. In addition to cohort studies, case-control studies are also used in epidemiological pharmacovigilance. Calculating the odds ratio (OR), they are faster and less expensive than cohorts, adapted to rare ADRs or those with a long latency period. They also make possible to study alongside the drug's other risk factors. Because of their retrospective nature, they can be affected by memory bias. They pose, as always in pharmacoepidemiology, the difficulty of the choice of controls. They are able to study the ADRs frequency higher than 1 per 10,000. Their role of alert turns out important in expectation of confirmation, sometimes long to come.

It should be emphasized that none of the pharmacoepidemiological methods (cohorts as well as case-control) allow establishing the causality between one drug and the occurrence of an ADR. Pharmacoepidemiology can only conclude on possible associations.

Other methods used are: file cross-referencing, capture/recapture method to truly know the incidence of drug-related ADRs, and database analysis with in particular the case/non-case method. It is also possible to couple these pharmacoepidemiologic results with the basic pharmacological properties of drugs, which helps to understand

and approach the mechanism of adverse drug effects. Thus, it has been possible to establish a relationship between serotonin 5-HT2C and histamine H1 receptors and antipsychotic-induced diabetes. These pharmacovigilance–pharmacodynamic studies allow not only to detect new ADRs but also to explain their mechanism(s).

A last source of information, recently identified, in pharmacovigilance is narrative of patients and consumers on Internet forums (blogs). These discussions may represent a new source of information and, despite their limitations, allow detect further alerts in pharmacovigilance.

4 Conclusion

PV and iatrogenic diseases are now important part of daily clinical practice in order to improve drug prescription. PV must bc taught to all health professional students, developed in hospital, clinics, and outpatient practice.

In fact, in front of any prescription, three reflexes should be automatic:

1. *"The pharmacological reflex"* which consists in defining the pharmacological and then the therapeutic class of the drug (s). This allows recalling the main expected pharmacodynamic effects and the main pharmacokinetic characteristics (cytochromes, route(s) of elimination, drug interactions…).
2. *"The pharmacovigilance reflex"* is necessary to systematically evoke a drug cause in front of any symptom or complaint from patients; it is the "iatrogenic reflex" which is illustrated by the sentence "What if it was the drug?" Think drug in front of any disease is a very useful attitude, allowing, for example, to avoid additional examinations often useless, expensive, and sometimes even dangerous.
3. *"The reporting reflex at the Pharmacovigilance Center"* in order to help future other prescribers and users of the drug(s) to a better and safe prescription.

Conflicts of Interest None.

Bibliography

Abou Taam M, Rossard C, Cantaloube I, Bouscaren N, Pochard L, Montastruc F, Montastruc JL, Bagheri H. Analyse of internet narratives on patient websites before and after benfluorex withdrawal and media coverage. Fundam Clin Pharmacol. 2012;26(Suppl 1):79.

Bagheri H, Lacroix I, Bondon-Guitton E, Damase-Michel C, Montastruc JL. Cyberpharmacovigilance: what is the usefulness of the social networks in pharmacovigilance? Therapie. 2016;71:241–4.

Baron JA, Sandler RS, Bresalier RS, Lanas A, Morton DG, Riddell R, Iverson ER, Demets DL. Cardiovascular events associated with rofecoxib: final analysis of the APPROVe trial. Lancet. 2008;372:1756–64.

Belton KJ. Attitude survey of adverse drug-reaction reporting by health care professionals across the European Union. The European Pharmacovigilance Research Group. Eur J Clin Pharmacol. 1997;52:423–7.

Bondon-Guitton E, Despas F, Becquemont L. The contribution of pharmacogenetics to pharmacovigilance. Therapie. 2016;71:223–8.

But TF, Cox AR, Oyebode J, Ferner RE. Internet accounts of survivors of serious adverse drug reactions: a study of experiences of Stevens Johnson syndrome and toxic epidermal necrolysis. Drug Saf. 2011;34:898.

Caillet C, Durrieu G, Jacquet A, Faucher A, Ouaret S, Perrault-Pochat MC, Kreft-Jaïs C, Castot A, Montastruc JL, French Network of Pharmacovigilance Centres. Safety surveillance of influenza A(H1N1)v monovalent vaccines during the 2009-2010 mass vaccination campaign in France. Eur J Clin Pharmacol. 2011;67(6):649–51.

Carpenter D, Zucker EJ, Avorn J. Drug-review deadlines and safety problems. N Engl J Med. 2008;358:1354–61.

Faillie JL. Case-non case studies: principles, methods, bias and interpretation. Therapie. 2018;73:247–55. pii: S0040-5957(17)30178-6.

Faillie JL, Montastruc F, Montastruc JL, Pariente A. Pharmacoepidemiology and its input to pharmacovigilance. Therapie. 2016;71:211–6.

Hazell L, Shakir SA. Under-reporting of adverse drug reactions: a systematic review. Drug Saf. 2006;29:385–96.

Hillaire-Buys D, Faillie JL, Montastruc JL. Pioglitazone and bladder cancer. Lancet. 2011;378:1543–4.

Lafond J. Pharmacovigilance implemented by patients: a necessity in the 21th century. Therapie. 2016;71:245–8.

Lagnaoui R, Moore N, Fach J, Longy-Boursier M, Begaud B. Adverse drug reactions in a department of systemic diseases-oriented internal medicine: prevalence, incidence, direct costs and avoidability. Eur J Clin Pharmacol. 2000;56:181–6.

Laroche ML, Batz A, Geniaux H, Fechant C, Merle L, Maison P. Pharmacovigilance in Europe: place of the Pharmacovigilance Risk Assessment Committee (PRAC) in organization and decisional process. Therapie. 2016;71:161–70.

Lazarou J, Pomeranz BH, Corey PN. Incidence of adverse drug reactions in hospitalized patients: a meta-analysis of prospective studies. JAMA. 1998;279:1200–5.

Lugardon S, Desboeuf K, Fernet P, Montastruc JL, Lapeyre-Mestre M. Using a capture-recapture method to assess the frequency of adverse drug reactions in a French university hospital. Br J Clin Pharmacol. 2006;62:225–31.

Miremont-Salamé G, Théophile H, Haramburu F, Bégaud B. Causality assessment in pharmacovigilance: the French method and its successive updates. Therapie. 2016;71:179–86.

Montastruc JL, Bagheri H, Geraud T, Lapeyre-Mestre M. Pharmacovigilance of self-medication. Therapie. 1997;52:105–10.

Montastruc JL, Sommet A, Lacroix I, Olivier P, Durrieu G, Damase-Michel C, Lapeyre-Mestre M, Bagheri H. Pharmacovigilance for evaluating adverse drug reactions: value, organization, and methods. Joint Bone Spine. 2006;73:629–32.

Montastruc F, Palmaro A, Bagheri H, Schmitt L, Montastruc JL, Lapeyre-Mestre M. Role of serotonin 5-HT2C and histamine H1 receptors in antipsychotic-induced diabetes: a pharmacoepidemiological-pharmacodynamic study in VigiBase. Eur Neuropsychopharmacol. 2015;25:1556–65.

Olivier P, Boulbes O, Tubery M, Lauque D, Montastruc JL, Lapeyre-Mestre M. Assessing the feasibility of using an adverse drug reaction preventability scale in clinical practice: a study in a French emergency department. Drug Saf. 2002;25:1035–44.

Pouyanne P, Haramburu F, Imbs JL, Begaud B. Admissions to hospital caused by adverse drug reactions: cross sectional incidence study. French Pharmacovigilance Centres. Br Med J. 2000;320:1036.

Smith Rogers A. Adverse drug events: identification and attribution. Drug Intell Clin Pharm. 1987;21:915–20.

Vial T. French pharmacovigilance: missions, organization and perspectives. Therapie. 2016;71:143–50.

Zed PJ, Abu-Laban RB, Balen RM, Loewen PS, Hohl CM, Brubacher JR, Wilbur K, Wiens MO, Samoy LJ, Lacaria K, Purssell RA. Incidence, severity and preventability of medication-related visits to the emergency department: a prospective study. CMAJ. 2008;178:1563–9.

Drug-Induced Gingival Overgrowth

Léa Bontemps, Frédérick Gaultier,
Fani Anagnostou, Anne-laure Ejeil,
and Sophie-Myriam Dridi

1　Introduction

Drug-induced gingival overgrowth (DGO) belongs to the group of iatrogenic gingival diseases with functional and aesthetic repercussions which can alter the quality of life. This periodontal disease was reported for the first time in 1939 as an adverse effect of phenytoin. Subsequently, gingival enlargement was attributed to other drugs.

The prevalence of this condition is difficult to assess. However, DGO is frequently observed,

L. Bontemps
Periodontology Department, Henri Mondor Hospital, APHP, Paris University, Paris, France
e-mail: lea.bontemps@parisdescartes.fr

F. Gaultier
Oral Medicine Surgery and Implantology Department, Henri Mondor Hospital, APHP, Paris University, Paris, France
e-mail: frederick.gaultier@parisdescartes.fr

F. Anagnostou
Periodontology Department, Pitié Salpêtrière Hospital, APHP, Paris University, Paris, France
e-mail: fani.anagnostou@univ-paris-diderot.fr

A.-l. Ejeil
Oral Medicine Surgery and Implantology Department, Bretonneau Hospital, APHP, Paris University, Paris, France
e-mail: anne-laure.ejeil@aphp.fr

S.-M. Dridi (✉)
Periodontology Department, Saint Roch Hospital, Nice Sophia Antipolis University, Nice, France
e-mail: dr.sm.dridi@free.fr

and beside epileptic patients, concerns an increasing number of patients with cardiovascular diseases or organ transplants.

Although the drugs involved have distinct pharmacological effects on their primary tissue targets, it appears that they act similarly on the gingival connective tissue. The pathogenesis of the lesions is partly related to an alteration of the homeostasis of the gingival connective tissue. However, the pathophysiological mechanisms leading to the development of gingival overgrowth are not yet fully understood.

Differential diagnosis is essential and requires appropriate multidisciplinary care.

The aim of this chapter is threefold:

- List the knowledge acquired concerning the pathogenesis of DGO.
- Present the clinical expression of this gingival disease and the clinical approach necessary for the differential diagnosis.
- Propose the therapeutic alternatives.

2　Etiopathogeny

2.1　Associated Drugs

The aetiology of gingival overgrowth involves three main drugs: phenytoin, some immunosuppressive agents, particularly cyclosporine, and the calcium channel blocking agents (Table 1).

© Springer Nature Switzerland AG 2021
S. Cousty, S. Laurencin-Dalicieux (eds.), *Drug-Induced Oral Complications*,
https://doi.org/10.1007/978-3-030-66973-7_2

Table 1 Estimated prevalence of DGO related to each drug. The heterogeneity in studies (inclusion criteria, evaluation criteria, and different studied populations) explains the significant differences in the results

	Pharmaceutic agent	Commercial name®	Prevalence of DGO		
			Dongari et al.	Brown et al.	Gawron et al.
Anticonvulsant	Phenytoin	Dihydan	50%	10–83%	70%
	Sodium valproate	Depakene	Rare		
	Phenobarbital	Gardenal	<5%		
	Vigabatrin	Sabril	Rare		
	Carbamazepine	Tegretol	–		
Immunosuppressant	Cyclosporine	Sandimmune Neoral	25–30% adult >70% child	7–80%	8–70%
Calcium channel blockers	Nifedipine	Adalat	6–15%	30–50%	15–83%
	Isradipine	Icaz	–		4%
	Felodipine	Flodil	Rare		21%
	Amlodipine	Amlor	Rare		
	Verapamil	Isoptin	<5%		
	Diltiazem	Tildiem	5–20%		

Derived from hydantoin, phenytoin is a non-sedative anti-seizure agent, known to induce an anticonvulsant activity, and is also prescribed to treat epilepsy and certain forms of neuralgia. It links with sodium channels and alters their conductance, thus inhibiting the onset of intense and repeated seizures. This explains its capacity to prevent tonic–clonic seizures (also called "the *grand mal* seizure disorder or epilepsy").

Introduced in the 1930s, its iatrogenic effect on the gingiva of patients treated with this drug was reported as early as 1939 by Kimball. Nowadays, it is no more prescribed as a first-intended medication and has been replaced by other specific drugs which are more efficient and initiate less side effects.

Produced from the fermentation of yeasts (*Trichoderma Polysporum* and *Cylindrocarpon Lucidum*), cyclosporine (also called cyclosporine A) was initially used in the 1970s as an antimicrobial agent. Its immunosuppressive properties were brought to light by Borel as soon as 1977; it initiates a specific inhibition of the immunocompetent lymphocyte activation; this inhibition leads to the suppression not only of the cell-mediated reaction but also of the T cell-dependent humoral response. It also inhibits the production of some lymphokines, particularly IL-2.

Thus, cyclosporine is currently administered to prevent rejection of organ transplants and also to treat rheumatoid polyarthritis, pemphigus, pemphigoid diseases, psoriasis, and atopic dermatitis. The occurrence of DGO in patients under cyclosporine has been reported in the early 1980s.

Calcium channel blockers are largely prescribed to prevent hypertension since 1978. These molecules link to the α1 subunit of the calcium channels, thus reducing the calcium flux entering the cell. Subsequently, they allow relaxation of the smooth muscles, vasodilatation, and decrease of blood pressure, on the one hand, and a decrease of the heart rate with a slower atrioventricular conduction time on the other hand.

In the literature, the two sub-classes of calcium channel blockers—dihydropyridines and non-dihydropyridines—are associated to the development of DGO, with a somehow higher prevalence for the dihydropyridines. The relationship between calcium channel blockers and DGO was first reported by Ramon in 1984.

2.2 Risk Factors

Patients treated with phenytoin, cyclosporine, and calcium channel blockers do not initiate systematic gingival overgrowth. This gingival pathology occurs at various degrees of severity and varies from one patient to another. The existence of an individual susceptibility towards the incriminated molecules is suspected and allows to distinguish

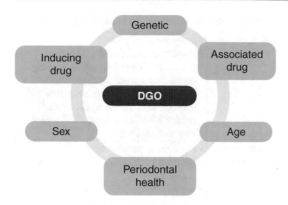

Fig. 1 DGO risk factors

"responders" and *"non-responders"* among the patients. This susceptibility could be related to the different ligand-receptor affinities and to the variations of cell ionic fluxes, the cell turn over rates, or the synthetic capacity of the cells.

Besides heredity, other risk factors have been reported (Fig. 1):

- Age: Prevalence and severity of lesions are higher in children and adolescents than in adults, especially for the anticonvulsants and for cyclosporine.
- Gender: Prevalence and severity are higher in males.
- The drug-related pharmacokinetic variables: Although the impact of treatment modalities remains unclear, it seems that a drug threshold concentration must be reached to initiate gingival changes, the concentration being specific to each patient.
- The associated drugs:
  - Prevalence of lesions increases when phenytoin is associated to other anticonvulsants.
  - Severity of lesions increases when cyclosporine is prescribed combined with a calcium channel blocker, which is a frequent combination to reduce the nephrotoxicity of cyclosporine.
  - Severity of lesions decreases if cyclosporine is prescribed combined with prednisolone or azathioprine.
- The presence of dental plaque and the patient's periodontal health status.

The important role of dental plaque as a cofactor in the development of gingival overgrowth is mentioned in the classification of periodontal diseases; DGOs are listed in the category of "plaque-induced gingival diseases and modified by medications." However, studies have some difficulty to determine whether dental plaque, mainly composed of bacterial biofilms, contributes to the development of DGOs, or if its accumulation is a consequence of the iatrogenic gingival changes; indeed, such lesions are also observed in patients with a high level of oral hygiene.

Nevertheless, it is reasonable to think that a plaque-induced inflammation exacerbates the clinical expression of DGO and this is true, whatever the incriminated drug. Moreover, when external plaque-retentive factors are present, such as orthodontic appliances, prevalence and severity of gingival overgrowth are increased. Several in vitro studies have attempted to support the relationship existing between the gingival inflammation and the severity of the gingival overgrowth, particularly via the implication of the pro-inflammatory cytokines; collagen synthesis, for example, is significantly increased when fibroblasts are co-cultured with nifedipine and IL-1β, compared to the group of fibroblasts and nifedipine alone. Secretion of IL-1β is increased in the presence of lipopolysaccharides (LPS) originating from the perio-pathogens. The involvement of IL-1β could therefore partly explain the existing relationship between the presence of dental plaque and the development of a drug-induced gingival overgrowth.

Many authors have also focused on the influence of the periodontal status prior to drug administration. In patients treated with cyclosporine, an existing periodontal disease prior to drug administration increases the risk to develop a severe DGO; similar results were obtained using other drugs. Inversely, strict oral hygiene programs proposed to patients under cyclosporine during the first 6 months following organ transplantation do not prevent the appearance of the lesions. Thus, prophylactic measures with an adequate plaque control allow to minimize the severity of gingival overgrowth but are not sufficient to prevent their occurrence.

In order to explain the variability of the gingival response to a same drug, the selection of some cell populations is one of the key issues. The existence, in the gingival connective tissue, the skin, and other organs, of functionally heterogeneous cell subpopulations is no more discussed. Indeed, healthy gingiva contains several subpopulations of fibroblasts which have different phenotypes. The clinical aspect and the histological characteristics of gingiva could reflect the presence of these fibroblast phenotypes which are more or less sensitive to the action of these drugs. This postulate is supported by in vitro studies which have demonstrated a change induced by phenytoin in the protein synthesis of some fibroblast strains. Despite this strong argument, there is no biological marker for the gingival fibroblast phenotype allowing to identify risk patients.

2.3 Physiopathological Mechanisms

The physiopathological mechanisms involved in DGO have not yet been totally elucidated. However, some studies have demonstrated a multifactorial aetiology: the molecule, the microbial gingival inflammation, and teeth.

The histological analysis of gingival biopsies shows, independently from the involved drug, an increase of the cell number and extracellular matrix (ECM) volume, probably resulting from a disturbed balance between synthesis activities and connective tissue degradation (Table 2).

Several authors have shown the critical role of cytokines and growth factors in the development of DGOs.

CTGF, EGF, IGF, PDGF, and TGF-β are considered as fibrosis markers as they stimulate the proliferation and synthesis of fibroblasts and subsequently the synthesis of collagen and other components of the extracellular matrix (ECM) (Fig. 2).

Both in vitro and in vivo studies have demonstrated that drugs involved in gingival overgrowth induce a stimulation of the expression and signalling pathways of these factors.

Under drug effect, the release of angiotensin II (Ang II) by the fibroblasts is increased, which induces the stimulation of the TGF-β expression. In the same way, the expression of endothelin-1

Table 2 Gingival manifestations associated with DGO

Epithelium	• Irregular parakeratosis • Protuberant epithelial ridges penetrating deep into the underlying connective tissue • Development of micro-abscesses (small foci of polymorphonuclear neutrophils) in the superficial layers of the epithelium
Connective tissue	• Fibroblasts proliferation • Increase in the number of collagen fibber bundles • Well-developed endoplasmic reticulum and moderate number of mitochondria: intense collagen synthesis • Increased amounts of extracellular matrix: proteoglycans, sulphated, and non-sulphated glycosaminoglycans, hexosamine, uronic acid • Increase of the vascular network and porosity • Chronic inflammatory infiltrate with predominance of plasma cells and lymphocytes

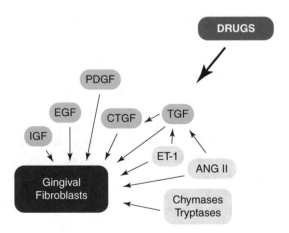

Fig. 2 Drug-activated growth factors and cytokines

(ET-1) is increased, thus allowing to stimulate fibroblast proliferation and modulate the synthesis of TGF-β.

Finally, an increase in the mastocyte degranulation process is observed, with an increased release of tryptase and chymase proteases, and a stimulation of the fibroblast and keratinocyte mitosis.

In addition to this stimulation of the signalling patterns, the inflammation process plays its role. In the presence of gingival inflammation—which is systematically associated to DGO—the production of the connective tissue components will increase, due to an increase of anabolism.

Along with this cell and molecular proliferation, the physiopathology of DGO includes a blocking effect on the degradation mechanisms via a disturbance in the calcium fluxes. Indeed, the three incriminated drugs induce the blocking of the cation channels and a subsequent decrease in the Ca^{2+} cytosolic levels (Table 3).

Collagen is degraded either by a phagocytosis mechanism or by collagenases. In the presence of phenytoin, cyclosporine, and nifedipine, a dose-dependent decrease of collagen phagocytosis by the fibroblasts is observed in vitro.

The first step in collagen phagocytosis relies on the interaction between collagen and fibroblasts The α-integrins play the role of surface receptors and their affinity for collagen is regulated by the Ca^{2+} cytosolic levels. The associated drugs, by disturbing the intracellular Ca^{2+} concentration, prevent an efficient phagocytosis by altering the affinity of the α-integrins and the link between collagen and its receptors.

The blocking of the cation channels also induces an inhibition of the active transport of folic acid through the cell membranes. Indeed, folic acid cell absorption depends upon two mechanisms: on the one hand, an active transport regulated by the cation channels, and on the other hand, a passive diffusion. The drug-induced disturbance of the calcium fluxes would thus induce a decrease in the absorption of folic acid by fibroblasts, leading to two negative effects: disturbance of the sulcular epithelium turnover and an impaired collagenase activation.

Table 3 Blocking of cation channels by the associated drugs

Phenytoin	Cyclosporine	Calcium channel blockers
• Membrane depolarization: inhibition of Ca^{2+} flux into excitable membranes	• Membrane depolarization: inhibition of Ca^{2+} flux into excitable membranes • Inhibition of Ca^{2+} uptake within gingival fibroblasts	• Inhibition of the L-type Ca^{2+} channel, inhibition of Ca^{2+} flux • Inhibition of Ca^{2+} uptake within gingival fibroblasts

Folic acid is used by the body particularly for the synthesis of pyrimidines and purines, and therefore DNA. A deficiency mainly affects cells with a high turn over: the DNA production is altered, mitosis becomes inefficient, and the maturation process is not achieved. Folic acid deficiency thus affects reversibly the sulcular epithelium maturation, consequently reducing the defence mechanisms of the gingiva against the bacterial inflammation.

This partly explains why DGO is rarely observed in edentulous areas where the connective tissue is protected by a thick keratinized epithelium, while in the dentulous areas, the sulcular epithelium which separates the connective tissue from the oral environment is thin and non-keratinized. Thus, any factor affecting the integrity of this epithelium renders the gingival tissue more susceptible to inflammation, and therefore to the deleterious effects of drugs.

The gingival fibroblasts synthetize matrix metalloproteinases (MMPs) involved in tissue remodelling via the ECM degradation. The cells also synthetize the inhibitors of these enzymes, the TIMPs (*tissue inhibitor of metalloproteinase*). The activation of collagenase is a complex process which depends on multiple biochemical pathways, involving the TIMPs and the MMPs and also the E-cadherins, SMAD, and AP-1 (Fig. 3).

E-cadherins and the SMAD activate the activator protein 1 (AP-1), which allows the inhibition of TIMP-1. The inhibition of TIMP-1 induces a decrease of the MMP-1 inhibition, which is required for collagenase activation.

It has been demonstrated that a decrease in the level of folic acid leads to a reduced expression of the E-cadherin and SMAD-4, and subsequently a disturbance in the chain previously described: MMP-1 is inhibited, the collagenase conversion into their active form is slowed, an imbalance then occurs enhancing anabolism and collagen fibrosis.

It is therefore possible to suggest a cause–effect relationship between the reduction of the cation flux by the three incriminated drugs, a reduced folic acid cell absorption, a disturbed collagenase activation, and a consequent dysfunction in connective tissue degradation. This hypothesis is supported by studies which have demonstrated:

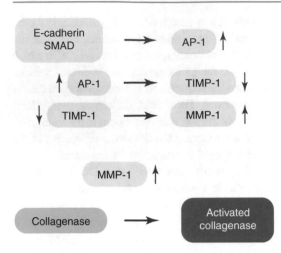

Fig. 3 Collagenase activation pathway

Table 4 Effects of folic acid in the treatment of DGO

Topical/ systemic	Results	Prevention/ reversal	Authors
Topical	Effective	Reversible effect	Drew et al. (1987)
Systemic	Effective	Reversible effect	Backman et al. (1989)
Systemic	Non-effective	Reversible effect	Brown et al.
Systemic	Effective	Prevention	Poppell et al. (1991)
Systemic	Effective	Prevention	Prasad et al. (2004)
Systemic	Effective	Prevention	Arya et al. (2011)

- A reduced gene expression of E-cadherin induced by the three drugs,
- Reduced levels of MMP-1 within the samples of hypertrophic gingiva, and
- Increased levels of TIMPs during the intake of cyclosporine and phenytoin.

A treatment option has even been suggested by some authors (Table 4). If the active transport of folic acid to the epithelial cells is blocked, the use of topical folic acid could allow to increase its extracellular concentration, in order to create a concentration gradient, and thus increase the fibroblast folic acid intake via a passive diffusion.

Furthermore, in vitro trials have shown a slower cell death process in the fibroblast population under the influence of these drugs. Nifedipine

limits on the one hand the cell death mechanisms by adherence, and on the other hand stops the nitrosative stress phenomenon, and subsequently cell death via apoptosis. As for cyclosporine, it has the capacity to inhibit molecules which induce apoptosis, such as Fas-L, caspases, and cytochrome C. The drugs would then have a protective effect against the apoptosis mechanisms, thus allowing subsequent fibroblast and extracellular matrix proliferation.

However, DGOs are not exclusively fibrous. Examination of human gingiva samples indeed shows that the nature of the gingival lesions is different according to the incriminated molecule; those induced by phenytoin are clearly the most fibrous ones, while those induced by cyclosporine are the most inflammatory, with a smaller proportion of fibrosis. As for nifedipine, it induces mixed lesions (Fig. 4).

Although the pathological mechanisms are still misknown, several hypothesis have been proposed to elucidate the predominance of the inflammatory component during a cyclosporine-induced gingival overgrowth; cyclosporine is a molecule which moreover has the potential to generate kidney and heart fibrosis.

The innate immune system is particularly developed within the oral cavity environment due to the numerous microbial and physical stimuli which do not exist in the kidney. Normally, this innate immune system is under a reciprocal regulation with the acquired immune system. However, cyclosporine inhibits the production of T lymphocytes stimulated by IL-2, which reduces the acquired immune response. The innate immune system could become very sensitive in the absence of the acquired immune system's "damping effect," when the latter is altered. In

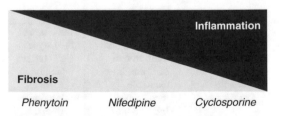

Fig. 4 Relationship between drugs, inflammation, and fibrosis

reaction, the innate immune response would become abnormally high, thus inducing the observed inflammatory phenomenon.

Moreover, cyclosporine inhibits cyclophilin, which consequently slows the production and maturation of collagen, via the inhibition of the prolyl-3-hydroxylase activity. Indeed, collagen hydroxylation on the proline remnants by the pro-lyl-3-hydroxylase (and the 4-hydroxylase) facili-tates the formation of the triple-helicoidal structure of collagen during its biosynthesis within the endoplasmic reticulum. Cyclosporine could have, via this pattern, an opposing effect on fibrosis.

On the other hand, assessment of the intra and extracellular presence of CTGF does not provide the same results depending on the drug. CTGF, considered as a marker for fibroblastic activity

and fibrosis, is observed at higher levels in the cases treated with phenytoin, compared to the other drugs. Inversely, during the intake of cyclo-sporine, CTGF is almost undetectable, with a severe increase of the inflammatory infiltrate.

Finally, in the presence of a cyclosporine-induced gingival overgrowth, the fibroblast syn-thesis of IL-6—pro-inflammatory cytokine—is increased. This increase may be due, at least par-tially, to the increased gingival inflammation in these patients, given that an inflammation pro-cess associated with the presence of LPS induces an increased IL-6 level.

The occurrence of drug-induced gingival overgrowth is therefore multifactorial and char-acterized by an imbalance between the synthesis and degradation mechanisms of the connective tissue components (Fig. 5).

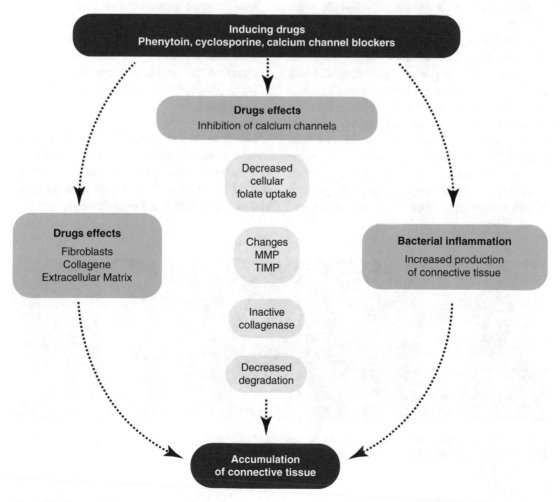

Fig. 5 DIGO mechanisms

3   Clinical Expression and Differential Diagnosis

3.1   Clinical Expression

Early changes in gingival morphology usually occur at 1–3 months after drug administration. However, gingival enlargement may be observed later. It usually begins with a papillary involvement: the papillae become oedematous and have a smooth or granular surface. Then, the enlargement spreads to the other sites of the gum, which becomes lobulated and even nodular, progressively reducing the height of the clinical crowns until these are completely covered in extreme situations. The enlargement predominantly affects the buccal and labial gingiva in the anterior regions of the mouth.

Most often, these clinical manifestations are similar from one drug to another and do not vary according to the offending molecule. However, exceptions are described in the literature, concerning especially phenobarbital and cyclosporine. In patients treated with phenobarbital, the gingiva grows globally and uniformly without lobulation of the papillae, and gingival lesions may be more severe in the posterior areas than in the anterior areas. If cyclosporine has been prescribed, the enlarged gingiva is markedly more inflammatory and the gingival bleeding is profuse. The development of small papillary and granular lesions on the surface of larger gingival lobulations is also often described (Fig. 6).

In general, gingival enlargement is not or slightly symptomatic and is accompanied by many functional signs of varying intensity:

- Dental displacements and secondary diastema are frequent because of the pressure exerted by the enlarged tissues on the teeth and cause speech and aesthetic impairment and
- Food stuffing is quite common, resulting in gingival sensitivities and halitosis. The latter is also favoured by the inexorable formation of gingival pockets, consequent to the increased volume of the gum, which results in an ineffective tooth brushing. Once formed, these pockets represent a privileged ecosystem for gram-negative anaerobic bacteria of the subgingival biofilms, which can at times exercise their deleterious activities on the periodontal tissues. The periodontal risk is therefore not negligible and the transition from gingivitis to periodontitis should be considered.

Similarly, if the patient is immunocompromised because of cyclosporine, the risk of chronic mycosis is possible. Gingival inflammation, by altering the mucosal barrier, promotes the penetration of Candida into the epithelial layers.

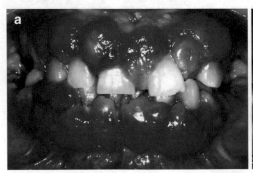 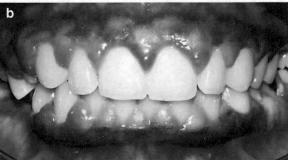

Fig. 6 Gingival overgrowth due to cyclosporine (**a**) and amlodipine (**b**). The presence of dental plaque worsens the gingival enlargement by generating an inflammatory process

3.2 Differential Diagnosis

An existing medication should not automatically direct the diagnosis towards an iatrogenic origin of the gingival overgrowth, for two reasons:

- Two gingival diseases can indeed coexist, might even worsen one another and
- The drugs incriminated in the gingival overgrowth do not systematically cause this type of lesion.

The differential diagnosis is therefore of primary importance; it eliminates other benign causes as well as proliferative syndromes and systemic pathologies, for which gingival overgrowth can be an inaugural manifestation.

Several points should be investigated during the clinical examination:

- Medical and dental history,
- Circumstances of occurrence, localization, and appearance of the lesions, and
- Symptoms and associated general signs.

Approximately ten aetiologies can lead to clinical manifestations similar to DGO (Table 5).

3.2.1 Malignant Diseases

Acute leukaemia is the most important malignant differential diagnosis; infiltration of gingival tissue by leukemic cells may cause a diffuse gingival overgrowth very similar to that induced by drugs (Fig. 7). The general condition of the patient is altered, and oral signs of anaemia, neutropenia, and thrombocytopenia may also be present. Acute myeloid leukaemia type 4 or 5 have a specific gingival tropism, which imposes the systematic prescription of a blood cell count.

Non-Hodgkin's lymphoma may present intraoral manifestations, which in most cases are tumours or ulcerations. Nevertheless, cases of papillary overgrowth have been reported. A biopsy and the absence of general signs allow this diagnosis elimination.

3.2.2 Benign Diseases

Bacterial gingivitis, when aggravated by an endocrine factor, can produce a pronounced and generalized enlargement (Fig. 8). Correction of risk factors, combined with periodontal therapy, can lead to remission.

In exceptional cases, an epulis may look like a diffuse tumour. A traumatic or hormonal factor must be sought out. The anatomopathological examination confirms the diagnosis (Fig. 9).

Plasma cells gingivitis is a rare immune response that may be similar to DGO, but unlike the latter, papillae are often decapitated (Fig. 10). As before, only the biopsy allows a definitive diagnosis.

Vitamin C deficiency may also be mentioned towards a gingival enlargement occurring in a malnourished patient, who shows an altered general condition as well as abnormalities of skin and appendages. In this case, the gingiva is particularly inflamed and haemorrhagic (Fig. 11).

Granulomatous diseases frequently lead to gingival overgrowth, including Crohn's disease (Fig. 12) and sarcoidosis; other mucosal lesions and systemic symptoms are then found. However, Wegener's granulomatosis, due to its pathognomonic "raspberry" gingival involvement, can be easily distinguished from DGO.

Hereditary gingival fibromatosis (Fig. 13) and neurofibromatosis type I (Fig. 14) also generate gingival enlargement. Thanks to their early diagnosis, patients are often aware of these two genetic diseases.

4 Therapeutic Care

Periodontal management should be instituted prophylactically before the medication begins, but this preventive measure is not always applied or applicable, depending on the patient's health. Therefore, most of the time, therapeutics are started once the gingival overgrowth is installed.

The first step is to institute an effective periodontal therapy. It comprises four steps, the third not being mandatory (Fig. 15). Its goal is to reduce the inflammatory component as well as

Table 5 Main differential diagnosis of DGO

	Lesion assessment	Functional assessment	Host assessment	Diagnostic criteria	Therapeutic care
Acute leukaemia	– Malignant gingival overgrowth – Acute evolution – Firm, fibrous, friable gingiva – Marked papillary injury	– Gingival pains $^{+/-}$ – Profuse gingival bleeding – Ulcerations, pallor, atypical dental pains $^{+/-}$, macrocheilia$^{+/-}$ – Fever – Firm/persistent lymphadenopathy – Alteration of the general condition: asthenia, anorexia, weight loss – Epistaxis, purpura, petechia, ecchymosis	– All ages – All populations	– Biopsy – Blood tests: pancytopenia, circulating blastosis *Specialized medical examination*	Hospital management (haematology service)
Non-Hodgkin lymphoma	– Malignant gingival overgrowth (Rare: a tumour aspect is more frequent) – Chronic evolution – Firm, fibrous gingiva	– Fever – Firm/persistent lymphadenopathy – $^{+/-}$ Alteration of the general condition: asthenia, anorexia, weight loss – Discomfort, night sweat – Pulmonary, pelvic, abdominal pains $^{+/-}$ – Cough $^{+/-}$	– All ages – All populations – General risk factors: autoimmune disease, immunosuppression, infections (EBV, HIV, HHV8), exposure to pesticides and radiations	Biopsy *Specialized medical examination*	Hospital management (haematology service)
Bacterial gingivitis aggravated by a risk factor	– Oedema, overgrowth – Chronic evolution – Soft and red gums – Plaque and calculus	– Dental mobility $^{+/-}$ – Induced or spontaneous gingival bleeding – Pain whenever an abscess is present, otherwise little or no pain	– All ages – All populations – Local risk factors: caries, braces, prosthesis, dental malposition, oral respiration, dry mouth – General risk factors: puberty, menstrual cycle, pregnancy, oral contraceptives, diabetes	None	– Periodontal care – Correction of local risk factors – Correction of general risk factors when possible (diabetes)

Gingival epulis	– Angiogranuloma: smooth, red pseudotumor. Ulceration +/_ Secondary fibrosis +/_ Acute evolution – Giant cells lesions: purple lobed exophytic tumour – Bone loss+/_	– Pains +/_ (secondary ulceration) – Profuse gingival bleeding – Dental mobility +/_ (Giant cells lesion)	– Angiogranuloma: women, young patients – All populations – Local risk factors: calculus, caries, braces, prosthesis – General risk factors: puberty, pregnancy (2nd trimester), diabetes	Biopsy	– Periodontal care – Surgical excision
Plasma cells gingivitis	– Oedema, overgrowth – Chronic evolution – Anterior areas – Firm, red gingiva – Papillary decapitation +/_ – Bone loss +/_	– Dental mobility +/_ – Induced or spontaneous gingival bleeding – Marked sensibility	– All ages – All populations – Local risk factors: exposure to an allergen	Biopsy	– Periodontal care – Surgical excision
Scurvy	– Benign gingival overgrowth – Chronic evolution – Red, oedematous gingiva – Bone loss +/_ (chronicity)	– Dental mobility (chronicity) – Spontaneous gingival bleeding – Petechia, purpura, ecchymosis – Dystrophic hair "corkscrew," alopecia – Lower limbs oedema	– All ages – All populations – General risk factors: malnutrition	– Food inquiry – Determination of vitamin C	Vitamin supplementation
Crohn's disease	– Benign gingival overgrowth – Chronic evolution – Firm, red, painless gingiva – Alteration of the entire gum height	– Gingival bleeding +/_ – Fissurous mucous ulcerations – Labial oedema +/_ – Fissurous cheilitis +/_ – Fever +/_ – Anorexia, weight loss +/_ – Abdominal pains, diarrhoea	– Teenagers/adults (15–40 years old) – Genetic susceptibility	– Biopsy – Blood tests: nutritional deficiencies, increased CRP *Specialized medical examination*	Hospital management (gastroenterology service)

(continued)

Table 5 (continued)

	Lesion assessment	Functional assessment	Host assessment	Diagnostic criteria	Therapeutic care
Sarcoidosis	– Benign gingival overgrowth – Chronic evolution – Firm, red, painless gingiva – Alteration of the entire gum height	– Induced or spontaneous gingival bleeding – Involvement of the salivary glands, the tongue, the palate$^{+/_-}$ – Fever $^{+/_-}$ – Lymphadenopathy – Weight loss $^{+/_-}$ – Dyspnoea$^{+/_-}$ – Chest pains, cough $^{+/_-}$	– Adults – All populations	Biopsy *Specialized medical examination*	Hospital management (internal medicine service)
Hereditary gingival fibromatosis	– Benign gingival overgrowth – Chronic evolution – Firm, non-haemorrhagic gingiva – Alteration of the entire gum height – Impacted and malpositioned teeth $^{+/_-}$	– Masticatory disorders $^{+/_-}$ – Elocution disorders $^{+/_-}$ – Possible hypertrichosis – Possible mental retardation	– Children (coincides with teeth eruption) – Family affliction$^{+/_-}$ – Isolated or associated with a syndrome	*Specialized medical examination*	– Periodontal care – Surgical excision in case of aesthetic/ functional disorders
Neurofibromatosis type 1	– Benign, unilateral gingival overgrowth – Chronic evolution – Firm, non-haemorrhagic gingiva – Dental eruption disorders$^{+/_-}$	– Neurofibroma – Pigment abnormalities (–– macules) – Skeletal disorders $^{+/_-}$	– All ages – All populations – Family affliction$^{+/_-}$ – Mutation of the neurofibromin gene (chromosome 17)	*Specialized medical examination*	Hospital management (internal medicine or dermatology service)

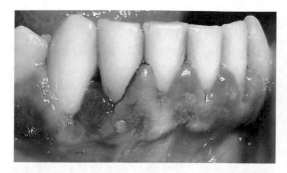

Fig. 7 Gingival overgrowth in acute leukaemia. (Courtesy of Dr N. Moreau—Paris Descartes)

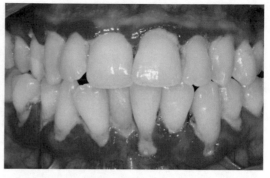

Fig. 10 Plasma cell gingivitis

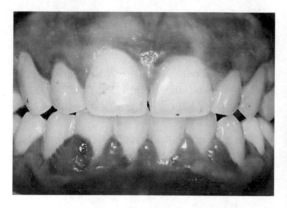

Fig. 8 Pregnancy gingivitis

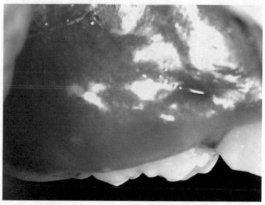

Fig. 11 Gingival overgrowth in scurvy. (Courtesy of Dr C. Joseph—Nice Sofia Antipolis)

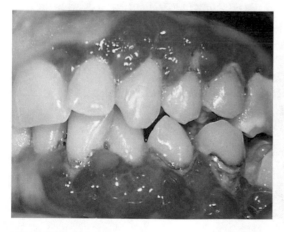

Fig. 9 Extended pregnancy epulis which did not regress after childbirth

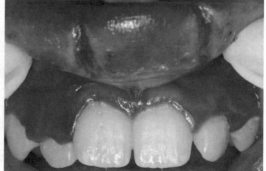

Fig. 12 Gingival overgrowth in sarcoidosis

restore and maintain the health, function, and aesthetics of the periodontium.

In case of an unsatisfactory tissue response to non-surgical periodontal therapy, i.e. the persis-
tence of an important fibrous component, it is appropriate to contact the physician, in order to change the iatrogenic medication by another specialty less deleterious for the periodontium—when it is possible.

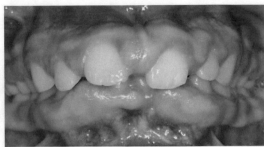

Fig. 13 Hereditary gingival fibromatosis

4.1   Therapeutic Education

This first step is essential; the patient acquires the skills he or she needs to best manage the side effects associated with his or her chronic illness. The point is to encourage good compliance and to facilitate the treatment contract. The clinical approach is simple and consists of explaining the medical basis of periodontal treatment and self-monitoring as many times as necessary and in a suitable manner.

4.2   Non-surgical Periodontal Treatment

Non-surgical periodontal treatment aims to control the infectious process induced by dental plaque. It includes:

- Teaching an effective oral hygiene technique.
- Brushing dental and gingival surfaces can be done with a manual or electric toothbrush, associated with a fluoride toothpaste to limit dental caries risk.
- Performing scaling or root planning in case of an attachment loss, in order to debride the gingival or periodontal pockets containing subgingival bacterial biofilms.

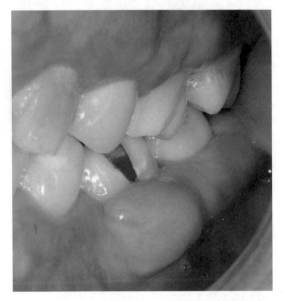

Fig. 14 Gingival overgrowth in neurofibromatosis type 1

Fig. 15 Main steps in the management of DGO

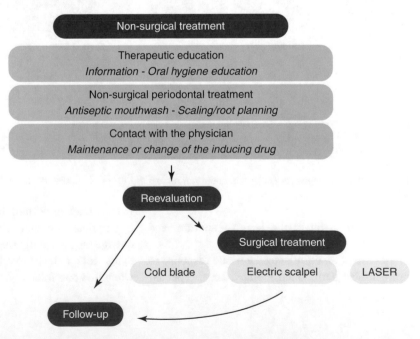

- Prescribing an alcohol-free antiseptic mouthwash based on 0.12% chlorhexidine throughout the treatment.
- This antiseptic, whose spectrum is perfectly suited to periodontal diseases, limits the inevitable intra-oral bacterial translocations and reduces the sensitivities generated by brushing thanks to its anti-inflammatory properties.
- The prescription of an antibiotic therapy for immunosuppression with cyclosporine.
- In addition, the prescription of an antibiotic therapy is necessary if severe periodontitis induced by dental plaque is associated with a gingival overgrowth of iatrogenic origin. In this latter situation, the periodontal pockets epithelium is completely disorganized and easily invaded by gram-negative anaerobic bacteria, which find suitable growing conditions in such a context.
- Two antibiotics are frequently indicated: metronidazole and azithromycin. The action of metronidazole (1.5–2 g/day for a minimum of seven days from the beginning of periodontal care) on subgingival biofilms is both quantitative and qualitative. However, this antibiotic is nephrotoxic has many side effects and modifies the hepatic metabolism of cyclosporine. Azithromycin seems to be more effective and does not interact with cyclosporine: a 3–5 days intake, with a dosage of 250–500 mg/day, appears to be sufficient in some cases. These positive effects would be linked to the particular structure of the molecule, which gives it an increased stability in an acid eco-system. Moreover, according to an animal study, azithromycin stimulates the phagocytic activity of fibroblasts, thus restoring the balance between collagen synthesis and degradation mechanisms.
- The prescription of an antifungal agent in association with the antibiotic therapy is necessary in case of mycosis concomitant with the bacterial infection, or of a susceptibility to this type of infection, in order to avoid the tissue penetration of pseudo filaments.
- The rehabilitation of iatrogenic dental cares and prostheses is crucial, as well as the elimination of dental irritating spines.

4.3 Periodontal Surgery

For severe forms of gingival overgrowth, surgery is often necessary because it is not always possible to obtain a satisfactory gingival morphology with the non-surgical therapy (Fig. 16).

The main operating difficulty is the management of bleeding, which is very marked due to the increased vascular network and permeability in the hypertrophic gingival tissue. Gingivectomy can be performed with a cold blade, an electric scalpel, or lasers (CO_2, Diode 810 nm) (Table 6).

The use of the cold blade has a double interest: the gingivectomy can be performed both in internal and external bevels, and a apically positioned flap of mixed thickness can be carried out at the end of intervention in order to decrease the depths of the vestibular periodontal pockets.

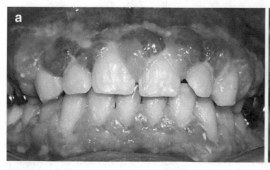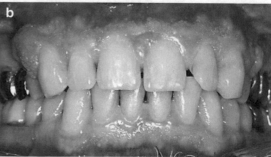

Fig. 16 Patient under cyclosporine and amlodipine. (**a**) Initial situation. (**b**) Situation after non-surgical periodontal treatment and replacement of amlodipine

Table 6 Pros and cons of cold blade, electric scalpel, and lasers for the management of DIGO

	Pros	Cons
Cold blade	• Clinical experience (1941) • Efficient and accurate section • Possibility to perform external and internal bevel gingivectomy at the same time • Possibility to perform an apically positioned flap • Good appreciation of the post-operative gingival contours (anterior areas)	• Intraoperative bleeding • Post-operative symptoms: oedema, pain, scarring • Long operative time
Electric scalpel	• Good management of haemostasis	• Thermal tissue necrosis: delayed healing • Post-operative symptoms: oedema, pain, scarring • Difficulty to change the gingival morphology, no possibility of moving the labial gingiva • Low clinical experience
LASER Diode 810 nm CO_2	• Good management of haemostasis • Efficient and accurate section • Formation of a blood clot suitable for healing • Sterilization of the surgical site • Reduction of post-operative symptoms: oedema, scarring • Reduction of the risk of recurrence at 6 months compared to the cold blade	• Difficulty to change the gingival morphology, no possibility of moving the labial gingiva • Cost and availability of equipment • Low clinical experience

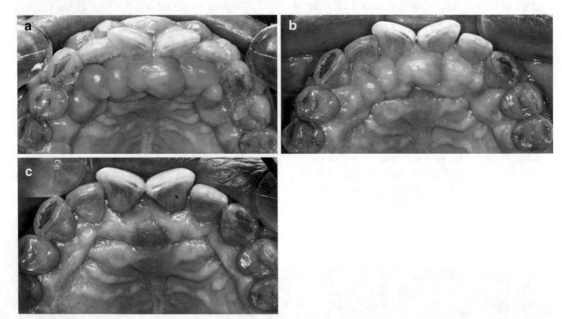

Fig. 17 Patient under cyclosporine and amlodipine. (**a**) Initial situation. (**b**) Situation after non-surgical periodontal treatment, without replacement of the treatment. (**c**) Situation after surgery, without replacement of the treatment (14 months' follow-up)

4.4 Periodontal Monitoring

No matter how severe the initial gingival overgrowth is, a periodic and individualized periodontal follow-up is an imperative condition to perpetuate the postoperative clinical situation obtained (Fig. 17).

5 Conclusion

Drug-induced gingival overgrowths are frequent periodontal lesions, for which treatment is difficult and requires a close collaboration with the physician.

The success of periodontal therapy imposes a clinical and scientific rigor. The plaque control should be done in a very assiduous way, the periodontal non-surgical therapy must be meticulous, and the choice of a surgical procedure has to be well thought out. The absence of gingival inflammation and the regularity of the long-term periodontal follow-up are important determinants to prevent recurrence, especially if the medications cannot be modified.

In addition, standardized studies are needed in order to better understand the cellular and molecular mechanisms involved in these gingival overgrowths, which will allow new preventive and curative therapeutic strategies.

Bibliography

Agrawal AA. Gingival enlargements: differential diagnosis and review of literature. World J Clin Cases. 2015;3(9):779–88.

Armitage GC. Development of a classification system for periodontal diseases and conditions. Ann Periodontol Am Acad Periodontol. 1999;4(1):1–6.

Asgary S, Aminzadeh N. Unilateral gingival enlargement in patient with neurofibromatosis type I. N Y State Dent J. 2012;78(6):50–3.

Aslangul E, Gadhoum H, Badoual C, Szwebel T, Perrot S, Le Jeunne C. A chronic gingival hypertrophy. Rev Med Interne. 2009;30(3):260–1.

Barclay S, Thomason JM, Idle JR, Seymour RA. The incidence and severity of nifedipine-induced gingival overgrowth. J Clin Periodontol. 1992;19(5):311–4.

Bekisz O, Darimont F, Rompen EH. Diffuse but unilateral gingival enlargement associated with von Recklinghausen neurofibromatosis: a case report. J Clin Periodontol. 2000;27(5):361–5.

Brown RS, Arany PR. Mechanism of drug-induced gingival overgrowth revisited: a unifying hypothesis. Oral Dis. 2015;21(1):e51–61.

Brown RS, Beaver WT, Bottomley WK. On the mechanism of drug-induced gingival hyperplasia. J Oral Pathol Med. 1991;20(5):201–9.

Calne RY, White DJ. The use of cyclosporin A in clinical organ grafting. Ann Surg. 1982;196(3):330–7.

Cole JA, Warthan MM, Hirano SA, Gowen CW, Williams JV. Scurvy in a 10-year-old boy. Pediatr Dermatol. 2011;28(4):444–6.

Coletta RD, Graner E. Hereditary gingival fibromatosis: a systematic review. J Periodontol. 2006;77(5):753–64.

Cotrim P, Martelli-Junior H, Graner E, Sauk JJ, Coletta RD. Cyclosporin A induces proliferation in human gingival fibroblasts via induction of transforming growth factor-beta1. J Periodontol. 2003;74(11):1625–33.

Dongari-Bagtzoglou A, Research, Science and Therapy Committee, American Academy of Periodontology. Drug-associated gingival enlargement. J Periodontol. 2004;75(10):1424–31.

Fujimori Y, Maeda S, Saeki M, Morisaki I, Kamisaki Y. Inhibition by nifedipine of adherence- and activated macrophage-induced death of human gingival fibroblasts. Eur J Pharmacol. 2001;415(1):95–103.

Gawron K, Łazarz-Bartyzel K, Potempa J, Chomyszyn-Gajewska M. Gingival fibromatosis: clinical, molecular and therapeutic issues. Orphanet J Rare Dis. 2016;11:9.

Gelfand EW, Cheung RK, Mills GB. The cyclosporins inhibit lymphocyte activation at more than one site. J Immunol. 1987;138(4):1115–20.

Graves DT, Li J, Cochran DL. Inflammation and uncoupling as mechanisms of periodontal bone loss. J Dent Res. 2011;90(2):143–53.

Güzel A, Köksal N, Aydın D, Aslan K, Gören F, Karagöz F. A rare clinical presentation of sarcoidosis; gingivitis. Oral Surg Oral Med Oral Pathol Oral Radiol. 2013;116(4):e280–2.

Hassell TM, Hefti AF. Drug-induced gingival overgrowth: old problem, new problem. Crit Rev Oral Biol. 1991;2(1):103–37.

Heasman PA, Hughes FJ. Drugs, medications and periodontal disease. Br Dent J. 2014;217(8):411–9.

Hou GL, Huang JS, Tsai CC. Analysis of oral manifestations of leukemia: a retrospective study. Oral Dis. 1997;3(1):31–8.

Iacopino AM, Doxey D, Cutler CW, Nares S, Stoever K, Fojt J, et al. Phenytoin and cyclosporine A specifically regulate macrophage phenotype and expression of platelet-derived growth factor and interleukin-1 in vitro and in vivo: possible molecular mechanism of drug-induced gingival hyperplasia. J Periodontol. 1997;68(1):73–83.

Ilgenli T, Atilla G, Baylas H. Effectiveness of periodontal therapy in patients with drug-induced gingival overgrowth. Long-term results. J Periodontol. 1999;70(9):967–72.

Joshi C, Shukla P. Plasma cell gingivitis. J Indian Soc Periodontol. 2015;19(2):221–3.

Jung J-Y, Jeong Y-J, Jeong T-S, Chung H-J, Kim W-J. Inhibition of apoptotic signals in overgrowth of human gingival fibroblasts by cyclosporin A treatment. Arch Oral Biol. 2008;53(11):1042–9.

Kantarci A, Cebeci I, Tuncer O, Carin M, Firatli E. Clinical effects of periodontal therapy on the severity of cyclosporin A-induced gingival hyperplasia. J Periodontol. 1999;70(6):587–93.

Khocht A, Schneider LC. Periodontal management of gingival overgrowth in the heart transplant patient: a case report. J Periodontol. 1997;68(11):1140–6.

Kimball O. The treatment of epilepsy with sodium diphenylhydantoinate. JAMA. 1939;112:1244–5.

Kwon JH, Song JC, Lee SH, Lee SY, Yang CW, Kim YS, et al. Non-Hodgkin's lymphoma manifest as gingival hyperplasia in a renal transplant recipient. Korean J Intern Med. 2005;20(4):330–4.

Lankarani KB, Sivandzadeh GR, Hassanpour S. Oral manifestation in inflammatory bowel disease: a review. World J Gastroenterol. 2013;19(46):8571–9.

Lederman D, Lumerman H, Reuben S, Freedman PD. Gingival hyperplasia associated with nifedipine therapy. Report of a case. Oral Surg Oral Med Oral Pathol. 1984;57(6):620–2.

Lim H-C, Kim C-S. Oral signs of acute leukemia for early detection. J Periodontal Implant Sci. 2014;44(6):293–9.

Lindhe J, Lang NP, Karring T. Plaque induced gingival diseases. In: Clinical periodontology and implant dentistry. 5th ed. Ames: Blackwell Munksgaard; 2008. p. 405–19.

Lucas RM, Howell LP, Wall BA. Nifedipine-induced gingival hyperplasia. A histochemical and ultrastructural study. J Periodontol. 1985;56(4):211–5.

Mavrogiannis M, Ellis JS, Seymour RA, Thomason JM. The efficacy of three different surgical techniques in the management of drug-induced gingival overgrowth. J Clin Periodontol. 2006b;33(9):677–82.

Mavrogiannis M, Ellis JS, Thomason JM, Seymour RA. The management of drug-induced gingival overgrowth. J Clin Periodontol. 2006a;33(6):434–9.

Maxymiw WG, Wood RE, Lee L. Primary, multi-focal, non-Hodgkin's lymphoma of the jaws presenting as periodontal disease in a renal transplant patient. Int J Oral Maxillofac Surg. 1991;20(2):69–70.

Mesa FL, Osuna A, Aneiros J, Gonzalez-Jaranay M, Bravo J, Junco P, et al. Antibiotic treatment of incipient drug-induced gingival overgrowth in adult renal transplant patients. J Periodontal Res. 2003;38(2):141–6.

Modéer T, Mendez C, Dahllöf G, Andurén I, Andersson G. Effect of phenytoin medication on the metabolism of epidermal growth factor receptor in cultured gingival fibroblasts. J Periodontal Res. 1990;25(2):120–7.

Moffitt ML, Bencivenni D, Cohen RE. Drug-induced gingival enlargement: an overview. Compend Contin Educ Dent. 2013;34(5):330–6.

Nagpal S, Acharya AB, Thakur SL. Periodontal disease and anemias associated with Crohn's disease. A case report. N Y State Dent J. 2012;78(2):47–50.

Nakou M, Kamma JJ, Andronikaki A, Mitsis F. Subgingival microflora associated with nifedipine-induced gingival overgrowth. J Periodontol. 1998;69(6):664–9.

Paik J-W, Kim C-S, Cho K-S, Chai J-K, Kim C-K, Choi S-H. Inhibition of cyclosporin A-induced gingival overgrowth by azithromycin through phagocytosis:

an in vivo and in vitro study. J Periodontol. 2004;75(3):380–7.

Raut A, Huryn J, Pollack A, Zlotolow I. Unusual gingival presentation of post-transplantation lymphoproliferative disorder: a case report and review of the literature. Oral Surg Oral Med Oral Pathol Oral Radiol Endod. 2000;90(4):436–41.

Savage NW, Daly CG. Gingival enlargements and localized gingival overgrowths. Aust Dent J. 2010;55(Suppl 1):55–60.

Seymour RA, Ellis JS, Thomason JM. Risk factors for drug-induced gingival overgrowth. J Clin Periodontol. 2000;27(4):217–23.

Spatafore CM, Keyes G, Skidmore AE. Lymphoma: an unusual oral presentation. J Endod. 1989;15(9):438–41.

Strachan D, Burton I, Pearson GJ. Is oral azithromycin effective for the treatment of cyclosporine-induced gingival hyperplasia in cardiac transplant recipients? J Clin Pharm Ther. 2003;28(4):329–38.

Subramani T, Rathnavelu V, Alitheen NB. The possible potential therapeutic targets for drug induced gingival overgrowth. Mediators Inflamm. 2013;2013: 639468.

Thomason JM, Seymour RA, Rice N. The prevalence and severity of cyclosporin and nifedipine-induced gingival overgrowth. J Clin Periodontol. 1993;20(1): 37–40.

Tipton DA, Stricklin GP, Dabbous MK. Fibroblast heterogeneity in collagenolytic response to cyclosporine. J Cell Biochem. 1991;46(2):152–65.

Trackman PC, Kantarci A. Molecular and clinical aspects of drug-induced gingival overgrowth. J Dent Res. 2015;94(4):540–6.

Uzel MI, Kantarci A, Hong HH, Uygur C, Sheff MC, Firatli E, et al. Connective tissue growth factor in drug-induced gingival overgrowth. J Periodontol. 2001;72(7):921–31.

Varga E, Lennon MA, Mair LH. Pre-transplant gingival hyperplasia predicts severe cyclosporin-induced gingival overgrowth in renal transplant patients. J Clin Periodontol. 1998;25(3):225–30.

Vogel RI. Gingival hyperplasia and folic acid deficiency from anticonvulsive drug therapy: a theoretical relationship. J Theor Biol. 1977;67(2): 269–78.

Williamson MS, Miller EK, Plemons J, Rees T, Iacopino AM. Cyclosporine A upregulates interleukin-6 gene expression in human gingiva: possible mechanism for gingival overgrowth. J Periodontol. 1994;65(10):895–903.

Wilson RF, Morel A, Smith D, Koffman CG, Ogg CS, Rigden SP, et al. Contribution of individual drugs to gingival overgrowth in adult and juvenile renal transplant patients treated with multiple therapy. J Clin Periodontol. 1998;25(6):457–64.

Wong W, Hodge MG, Lewis A, Sharpstone P, Kingswood JC. Resolution of cyclosporin-induced gingival hypertrophy with metronidazole. Lancet Lond Engl. 1994;343(8903):986.

Drug-Induced Oral Mucosal Pigmentation

Henri Tenenbaum, Catherine Petit, and Olivier Huck

1   Introduction

Oral mucosal pigmentation is a common clinical finding appearing as focal or diffuse lesions that may be physiological (racial or ethnic pigmentation), induced by endogenous pigments (melanin, haemoglobin, hemosiderin or carotene) and by exogenous materials (such as amalgam). Melanin is produced by melanocytes in the basal layer of the epithelium and is transferred to adjacent keratinocytes via membrane-bound organelles called melanosomes. Nevus cells that are derived from the neural crest and are found in the skin and mucosa also synthesize melanin. Pigmented lesions induced by increased melanin deposition may be brown, blue, grey or black, depending on the amount and location of melanin.

Physiologic pigmentation is related to ethnicity and predominantly found in dark-skinned populations. These pigmentations are usually bilateral and found in gingival and buccal mucosa.

Pathologic processes in the oral mucosa can be associated with some systemic diseases. Systemic diseases such as Peutz–Jeghers syndrome, Laugier–Hunziker syndrome, Addison's disease and some other rare diseases, such as polyostotic fibrous dysplasia, Nelson syndrome and hyper-thyroidism, are associated with oral melanotic pigmentation. Deposition of melanin in the connective tissue may also be found after tobacco smoking (smoker's melanosis) and long-standing inflammation in conditions such as oral lichen planus, pemphigus and pemphigoid.

Localized mechanical, physical and chemical stimuli may have an additional effect on pigmentation of the oral mucosa. Chronic irritation may occasionally result in the development of oral melanoacanthoma.

Drug-induced adverse reactions in the oral mucosa vary with the drug and its pharmacodynamics and pharmacokinetics, as well as any individual variability in drug metabolism. Pigmentary modifications in the oral mucosa may be induced by different medications, including anti-malarial drugs (chloroquine phosphate, hydroxychloroquine, quinidine, quinacrine), tranquilizers (chlorpromazine), chemotherapeutics (doxorubicin, busulfan, bleomycin, cyclophosphamide, clofazimine, imatinib), anti-retroviral agents (zidovudine, azidothymidine, ketoconazole), antibiotics (tetracyclines, minocycline) and laxatives (phenolphthalein).

The clinical aspect of abnormal oral mucosal pigmentation is a challenge for the clinician to accurately diagnose. The dental practitioner should have a thorough understanding of the aetiology of oral mucosal lesions and pigmentation. He must be able to guide the diagnosis and to refer to specialist services if necessary.

H. Tenenbaum (✉) · C. Petit · O. Huck
Dental Faculty, University of Strasbourg, Strasbourg, France

© Springer Nature Switzerland AG 2021
S. Cousty, S. Laurencin-Dalicieux (eds.), *Drug-Induced Oral Complications*,
https://doi.org/10.1007/978-3-030-66973-7_3

2   Aetiology of Oral Pigmentation

Causes of oral pigmentation are numerous. Pigments associated with mucosal discoloration could be classified as endogenous (melanin, haemoglobin, hemosiderin, carotene) and exogenous (metals and drug-related pigments).

Kauzman et al. have proposed a classification based on the distribution of the pigmentation (Fig. 1).

2.1   Physiological Oral Pigmentation

Oral mucosal pigmentation is closely associated with ethnicity. Physiological pigmentation is frequent in Asians, Africans and Mediterranean people, usually presenting as multifocal or diffuse, bilateral, light to dark brown macules on the gingiva and mucosa of the hard palate. The degree of gingival pigmentation is directly related to skin pigmentation. In light-skinned individuals, gingiva is mainly non-pigmented but in dark-skinned people pigmented gingiva is extremely frequent.

The colour change of the oral mucosa could be due to accumulation of one or more pigments in tissues and is generally more pronounced in the anterior regions of the mouth. This increase in pigmentation is due to increase in melanocyte activity and not due to a greater number of melanocytes. The described tends to increase in both intensity and surface area with increasing age but is not always obvious (Figs. 2a, b and 3).

2.2   Endogenous Oral Pigmentation

2.2.1   Systemic Diseases

Pigmentation associated with systemic disease, such as Peutz–Jeghers syndrome, Laugier–Hunziker syndrome, Albright syndrome, Addison's disease and neurofibromatosis, occurs as "*Café au lait*" macules or diffuse pigmentation involving mucosa and skin.

Peutz–Jeghers syndrome is a rare autosomal dominant inherited disorder characterized by intestinal hamartomatous polyps in association with a distinct pattern of skin and mucosal macular melanin deposition. Patients with Peutz–Jeghers syndrome have a 15-fold increased risk of developing intestinal cancer compared with the general population. In Peutz–Jeghers syndrome, it is suggested that the pigmented lesions develop secondary to the mutation of the LKB1

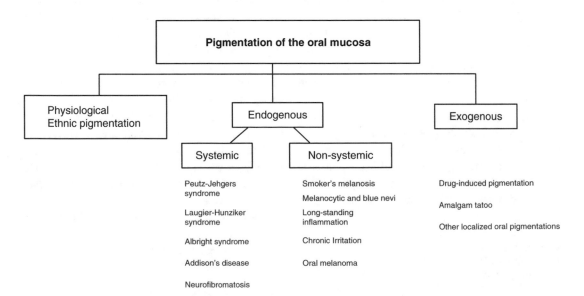

Fig. 1 Classification of oral pigmentations

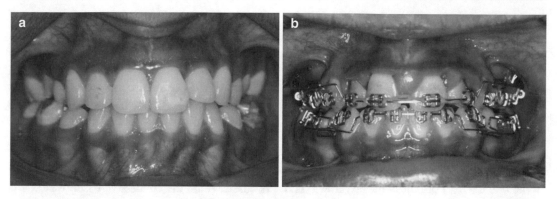

Fig. 2 (**a**) Physiological ethnic pigmentation in a 16-year-old North African woman. (**b**) Same pigmentation 20 years later

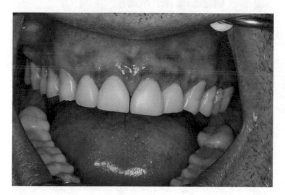

Fig. 3 Physiological ethnic pigmentation in the anterior area

gene, which activates the Wnt/b catenin pathway and contributes to the stimulation of melanocytes, thereby causing the excess production of melanin.

Laugier–Hunziker syndrome is a rare acquired disorder characterized by diffuse hyperpigmentation of the oral mucosa and longitudinal melanonychia in adults. The macular lesions have less than 5 mm in diameter. Laugier–Hunziker syndrome is considered to be a benign disease with no systemic manifestation or malignant potential.

Albright syndrome (also called McCune-Albright syndrome) is a rare genetic disorder of bones, skin and mucosal pigmentation and hormonal problems with premature sexual development. GNAS1 gene mutation and cAMP-mediated tyrosine kinase activation in melanocytes may play important roles in the formation of pigmented lesions in Albright syndrome.

Addison's disease is characterized by a primary adrenocortical insufficiency with decreased cortisol and aldosterone production, stimulating the expression of ACTH. Symptoms generally come on slowly and may include abdominal pain, weakness and weight loss. Hyperpigmentation of the skin and/or the oral mucosa in certain areas may also occur.

The pathophysiologic mechanism of pigmentation in neurofibromatosis remains uncertain.

In all these conditions, melanin pigment in the basal cell layer of the skin and/or oral mucosa increases with incontinent melanin and melanophages in the lamina propria to varying degrees, without concomitant deposition of iron unless there has been haemorrhage.

2.2.2 Smoker's Melanosis

Smoking may induce oral pigmentation in light-skinned individuals and accentuate the pigmentation of dark-skinned patients. Smoker's melanosis occurs in up to 21.5% of smokers. Women are more commonly affected than men, suggesting a possible synergistic effect between female sexual hormones and smoking. The intensity of the pigmentation is related to the duration and amount of smoking. There is an increased production of melanin that may provide a biologic defence against the noxious agents present in tobacco smoke. The brown-black lesions most often involve the anterior labial gingiva, followed by the buccal mucosa. Smoker's melanosis usually disappears within 3 years of smoking cessation. A biopsy should be performed if there is surface elevation or increased pigment intensity, or if the pigmentation appears in an unexpected site. There is no evidence supporting the malignant transformation of smoker's melanosis, but caution should be taken about other systemic complications associated with smoking. Smoker's melanosis can be used as a clinical finding to identify the smoking history.

2.2.3 Melanocytic and Blue Nevi

In the oral cavity, both melanocytic (brown) and blue nevi are rare with the hard palate being the site of predilection. Histologically, nevi are composed of an accumulation of nevus cells in the basal epithelial layers, the connective tissue or both. As such, they are classified as junctional, intradermal or intramucosal and compound nevi. Junctional nevi are flat and dark brown in colour because the nevus cells proliferate at the tips of the rete pegs close to the surface. Intramucosal and compound nevi are typically light brown, dome-shaped lesions. Blue nevi are characterized by proliferation of dermal melanocytes within the deep connective tissue at some distance from the surface epithelium, which accounts for the blue colour. Buchner et al. stated that intramucosal nevi are the most common type and are seen most frequently on the buccal mucosa. The blue nevus is the second most common type, occurring most commonly on the palate. It may be difficult to differentiate clinically between a nevus and an early lesion of mucosal melanoma, especially in the palate, the most common site for both lesions. Although transformation of oral pigmented nevi to melanoma has not been well documented, probably in relation of the rarity of reported lesions, it is believed that nevi may represent precursor lesions to oral mucosal melanoma. It is therefore recommended to completely excise these lesions and submit it for histopathologic examination.

2.2.4 Long-Standing Inflammation

Post-inflammatory hypermelanosis has also been described in the literature. Following chronic inflammatory states present in the oral tissues, such as that induced by lichenoid reactions and lichen planus, excess deposits of melanin develop in the epithelial basal layer and surrounding connective tissue of the oral mucosa. The development of a post-inflammatory pigmentation may include two different processes: an increase in melanin production related to a direct stimulation of melanocytes by inflammatory mediators, and an abnormal distribution of melanin pigment.

Macrophages laden with melanin (melanophages) could be detected in the connective tissue underlying epithelium. Melanin is probably released within the connective tissue where it is phagocytized by melanophages.

2.2.5 Chronic Irritation

Localized traumatic pigmentation can be due to injuries contaminated by foreign material (dust). Trauma could also result in oral melanoacanthoma which is an uncommon benign-pigmented lesion of the oral mucosa, characterized by proliferation of dendritic melanocytes dispersed throughout the thickness of an acanthotic and hyperkeratotic surface epithelium. Clinically, the lesion appears hyperpigmented black or brown, flat or slightly raised. This lesion, in contrast to most of other benign-pigmented lesions, has a tendency to enlarge rapidly, which raises the possibility of a malignant process. However, its tendency to occur in young black females distinguishes it from melanoma, which is uncommon in this age and racial group. Goode et al. stated that the buccal mucosa is the most common site of occurrence, which may be related to greater frequency of trauma in this area. Oral melanoacanthoma appears to be a reactive lesion with no malignant potential. In some cases, the lesion disappears after incisional biopsy or removal of the offending stimulus.

2.2.6 Oral Melanoma

Oral mucosal melanoma is as uncommon as oral melanoacanthoma, accounting for less than 1% of all oral malignancies. Oral melanomas account for 0.2–8% of all melanomas in the United States and Europe, but for 11–12.4% of all melanomas in Japan. Although occurrence of cutaneous melanomas is less common in dark-skinned races, these races have a greater relative incidence of oral mucosal melanomas. Oral melanoma is diagnosed with a greater incidence in men than women. The palate is the most common site, representing about 40% of cases, and gingiva accounting for 33% of cases. Oral mucosal melanomas are characterized by proliferation of malignant melanocytes either along the junction between the epithelium and connective tissue or deep inside the connective tissue. Clinically, oral melanoma may appear as an asymptomatic, slowly growing brown or black patch with asymmetric and irregular borders or as a rapidly enlarging mass associated with ulceration, bleeding, pain and bone destruction. A few oral melanomas are non-pigmented (amelanotic). Although oral mucosal melanomas are rare, they represent a serious and often fatal disease. Oral mucosal melanoma tends to be more aggressive than its cutaneous counterparts and is mostly presented at a later stage of the disease.

2.3 Exogenous Oral Pigmentation

2.3.1 Drug-Induced Pigmentation

Adverse-drug effects commonly affect the oral mucosa. Pathologic changes in the oral mucosa can be associated with several drugs (Table 1). These adverse reactions depend on the drug and its pharmacodynamics and pharmacokinetics, as well as any individual variability in drug metabolism. Pigmentary modifications in the oral mucosa may be induced by many medications, including anti-malarial drugs (chloroquine phosphate, hydroxychloroquine, quinidine, quinacrine), tranquilizers (chlorpromazine), chemotherapeutics (imatinib, bleomycin, clofazimine, doxorubicin, busulfan, cyclophosphamide), anti-retroviral agents (zidovudine, azidothymidine, ketoconazole), antibiotics (tetracyclines, minocycline), anti-epileptics (retigabine) and laxatives (phenolphthalein).

Medication-associated pigmentation of the oral cavity is induced by: (a) pigmented breakdown products of the drug itself; (b) drug metabolites chelated with iron or (c) drugs that are able to induce melanin formation (phenolphthalein).

Anti-malarial agents, such as chloroquine diphosphate and hydroxyl chloroquine sulphate,

Table 1 Drugs associated with oral mucosal pigmentation

Antimalarials:
Chloroquine phosphate
Hydroxychloroquine
Quinidine
Quinacrine
Tranquilizers:
Chlorpromazine
Chemotherapeutics:
Doxorubicin
Busulfan
Bleomycin
Cyclophosphamide
Imatinib
Clofazimine
Anti-retroviral agents:
Zidovudine
Azidothymidine
Ketoconazole
Antibiotics:
Tetracycline
Minocycline
Laxatives:
Phenolphthalein
Anti-epileptics:
Retigabine

are administered for the treatment of several dermatologic and rheumatologic disorders. They possess anti-inflammatory or immunosuppressive functions, and they are known to induce hyperpigmentation of the oral mucosa via the complex interaction of drug metabolites, iron and/or melanin. Systemic administration of these drugs for a prolonged period is responsible for the appearance of multifocal hyperpigmentation, which is reversible once the medication is discontinued. Oral pigmentation secondary to drug therapy can be attributed to the stimulation of melanin production by melanocytes and/or the deposition of metabolic products of the drugs in the tissues.

Imatinib (imatinib mesylate, brand names Gleevec or Glivec) used in the treatment of certain cancers, including chronic myeloid leukaemia (CML), is a tyrosine kinase inhibitor that impairs the constitutively active tyrosine kinase BCR-ABL. The Food and Drug Administration has approved it in 2001 for the treatment of

CML. It blocks the activity of the mutated BCR-ABL tyrosine kinase of CML. In addition, imatinib blocks the binding of ligands to c-kit receptors on melanocytes, reducing the activity of melanocytes and leading to hypopigmentation. Imatinib is more commonly associated with skin hypopigmentation, but in recent articles, patients on imatinib were noted to develop diffuse hyperpigmentation on the hard palate. The diagnosis of imatinib-related pigmentation depends on a thorough medical history and characteristic clinical features. The hyperpigmented lesions are benign, and no treatment is required.

Clofazimine, a potent anti-inflammatory drug for treating leprosy, has red metabolites, which may lead to mucosal pigmentation.

Conjugated oestrogen has also been reported to induce oral pigmentation by lowering the plasma concentration of cortisol and stimulating adrenocorticotrophic hormone (ACTH) production. ACTH and alpha-melanocyte–stimulating hormone (a-MSH) are both the post-translational processing derivatives of pro-opiomelanocortin (POMC) products, with a-MSH being the first 13 amino acids of ACTH; as such, elevated levels of ACTH automatically increase the expression of a-MSH, thus resulting in hypermelanosis.

Chloroquine and other quinine derivatives are used in the treatment of malaria, cardiac arrhythmia and a variety of immunologic diseases including systemic and discoid lupus erythematous and rheumatoid arthritis. Mucosal discoloration associated with these drugs mostly involves the hard palate only and appears as blue-grey or blue-black in colour.

Tetracyclines, and especially minocycline, could be used in the long-term treatment of refractory acne vulgaris. It can cause pigmentation of the oral mucosa that is due to staining of the underlying alveolar bone and not as a consequence of an increased presence of melanin in the mucosa. The alveolar bone can be seen through the thin overlying oral mucosa (especially the maxillary anterior alveolar mucosa) as a grey discoloration.

Retigabine, a therapy used for the management of drug-resistant epilepsy, is the first available neuronal potassium channel opening drug. It acts to improve the stability of neurones, subsequently preventing seizures. The results obtained with retigabine in phase III regulatory trials have been positive in the clinical management of refractory epilepsy. However, significant side effects associated with retigabine have resulted in the European Medicine Agency (EMA), to recommend retigabine as a last resort therapy. This recommendation is primarily a result of the pigmentation (a blue-purple coloration) of the skin, nails, lips, oral (hard palate) mucosa and eye tissues that can develop following its use. The mechanism in which this pigmentation is induced is as yet unknown. Recent studies in rats have implicated pigmented dimerization products of retigabine in producing the discolouration. The histopathological features reported in a biopsy sample of dyspigmented mucosa of the hard palate by Shkolnik et al. showed normal epithelium without any melanin pigmentation.

2.3.2 Amalgam Tattoo

Deposition of dental amalgam within the tissues, known as an amalgam tattoo, is one of the most common aetiology of exogenous oral mucosal pigmentation. Clinically, it appears as a localized flat, blue-black asymptomatic lesion of variable dimensions. No signs of inflammation are present at the periphery of the lesion. The pigmentation is induced by different mechanisms, including mechanical penetration into soft tissues, corrosion phenomena and release of metallic components. Amalgam and its metal components (silver, mercury and tin) can be found in the oral mucosa during dental treatment with rotating instruments and the placement of dental restorations, or at the time of tooth extraction. If it is found next to a large amalgam restoration, it is easily recognizable.

Amalgam consists of three phases: phase γ ($SnAg_3$), phase $\gamma 1$ (Hg_3Ag_2) and phase $\gamma 2$ (Sn_8Hg), with phase $\gamma 2$ being the most corrodible. These phases have different degradation patterns, so they do not contribute equally to pigmentation. Phase $\gamma 2$ is degraded rapidly and does not participate in pigmentation. Phase $\gamma 1$ degrades slowly, with loss of Hg but there is no Hg in the pigment. Phase γ is the slowest to degrade and is responsible for the pigmentation, persisting as Ag in granular form, and sulphur particles. Ag becomes fixed to basal membranes, in collagen and elastic fibres and the perineuria, or may be phagocytized by macrophages, being the only remaining component. Sn is lost by corrosion.

A radiograph may reveal the presence of amalgam particles in the soft tissues, but this is not the case in about 75% of individuals where the metal is widely dispersed and the particles too small. Although all three phases of amalgam are radiopaque, the radiopacity of phase γ may disappear by fragmentation and dispersion within 1 year. This explains the lack of radiopacity in many pigmentations and their possible confusion with melanosis.

In case of doubt, a biopsy should be performed to demonstrate the presence of amalgam particles in the connective tissue and exclude melanocytic lesions. Identifying dark brown/grey particles, often aligned along collagen fibres and rarely associated with a foreign body–type immune reaction, makes the histologic diagnosis.

Embedded graphite from pencil may mimic an amalgam tattoo. The lesion occurs most frequently in the anterior palate of young children, appearing as an irregular grey to black macule (Fig. 4). Systemic ingestion of lead or bismuth can also induce oral mucosal pigmentation.

2.3.3 Other Exogenous Oral Pigmentations

Orthodontic brackets and arch wires include various proportions of nickel (Ni), copper (Cu), titanium (Ti), cobalt (Co) and chromium (Cr). Metallic ions can be released from these appliances and later be identified within the oral mucosa.

The silver solder joining the bracket to the arch wire of the orthodontic appliance may also be released and be detected in the oral soft tissues. It is unlikely that the silver was "tattooed" or implanted in a similar fashion to an amalgam tattoo. The silver solder could undergo electrolytic corrosion in the presence of salivary enzymes and bacteria in the gingival sulcular biofilm, as has been demonstrated by Joska et al. in relation to Ag in cast post and core restorations. Soluble silver ions present in the gingival sulcus of a molar tooth enclosed by a bracket could penetrate the gingival epithelium and subsequently form insoluble precipitates in the gingival tissues with sulphur derived from cellular sulphur-containing enzymes. This situation is similar to what occurs in systemic argyrosis, where ingested silver is absorbed in the small intestine and transferred through the blood as soluble colloids or salts and later deposited in various tissues where it is reduced to the metallic form. There it forms insoluble silver sulphide in conjunction with S from cellular enzymes and produces blue-grey skin pigmentation.

Metallic and metal-ceramic reconstructions may also induce gingival pigmentations (Fig. 5).

An association between habitual khat chewing and mucosal pigmentation has been suggested. Khat, or qat (*Catha edulis*), is a shrub indigenous

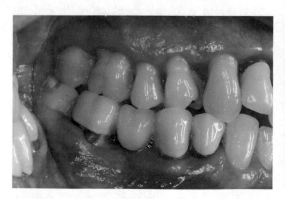

Fig. 4 Embedded graphite pigmentation

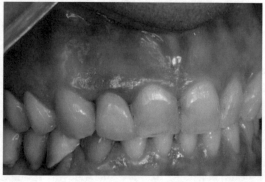

Fig. 5 Exogenous pigmentation in relation with the metal-ceramic crown on tooth 12

to Yemen and certain parts of eastern Africa. Ashri and Gazi described a single case where mucosal pigmentation was noted on the gingiva, buccal mucosa and tongue, with scattered patches of darker brown areas on the vestibular regions of a khat chewer.

3   Differential Diagnosis

Oral pigmentation has a variety of causes that must be fully considered by the diagnosing clinician, and any underlying disease or malignancy should be carefully checked.

Oral pigmentations could be focal, multifocal or diffuse. They may be black, grey, blue, purple or brown in colour. They may be flat or swollen. They can be localized accumulations of melanin, hemosiderin, and exogenous metal, or some are even indications of an internal disease. The differential diagnosis can be lengthy in certain conditions with multiple and complex lesions with pigmentations. Evaluation of a patient presenting with an oral pigmented lesion should include a full medical and dental history, extraoral and intraoral examinations and laboratory tests. The history should include the onset and duration of the lesion, the presence of associated skin hyperpigmentation, the presence of systemic signs and symptoms (e.g., discomfort, tiredness, weight loss), use of medications and smoking habits. Pigmented lesions on the face, perioral skin and lips should be noted. The number, distribution, size, shape and colour of intraoral-pigmented lesions should be assessed. In general, benign-pigmented lesions are small, symmetric and uniform in colour, with regular borders. They may be either flat or slightly elevated. In contrast, irregular borders, colour variation and surface ulceration suggest malignancy. Clinical tests such as diascopy and radiography and laboratory investigations such as blood tests can be used to confirm a clinical impression and reach a definitive diagnosis. Although biopsy is a helpful aid to diagnosis for localized lesions and is usually recommended to exclude melanocytic lesions, the more diffuse lesions will require a thorough history and laboratory studies in order to make a definitive diagnosis. Even though only a few lesions are reported to undergo malignant transformation, the limited data regarding malignancy transformation in oral lesions cannot be simply ruled out.

4   Treatment

No active treatment is required to manage most cases presenting oral pigmentation.

In front of a smoker's melanosis, the management requires to present to the patient the benefits of smoking cessation and to advise him to consult a physician or an anti-smoking centre.

When inflammatory pathologies or chronic irritations have induced oral pigmentations, these potential causes must be eliminated. In the case of drug-induced pigmentations, it is advisable to get in touch with the attending physician to consider substitutes if possible. Amalgam tattoos require care only if they are accompanied by aesthetic damage. Then, the treatment will be a surgical removal.

5   Conclusion

The diagnostic procedure of pigmented lesions of the oral cavity is quite challenging. Clinicians can make the diagnosis on clinical grounds alone. Histological evaluation of oral pigmentation is often required for a definitive diagnosis. We have tried to highlight the different oral-pigmented lesions that clinicians can most possibly come across during a routine check-up of the patients in order to help them to differentially diagnose oral-pigmented lesions and improve their understanding to differentiate between normal and diseased conditions.

Bibliography

Ashri N, Gazi M. More unusual pigmentation of the gingiva. Oral Surg Oral Med Oral Pathol. 1990;70(4):445–9.

Axell T, Hedin CA. Epidemiologic study of excessive oral melanin pigmentation with special reference to the influence of tobacco habits. Scand J Dent Res. 1982;90:434–42.

Barker BF, Carpenter WM, Darniels TE, et al. Oral mucosal melanomas: the WESTOP Banff workshop proceedings, Western Society of Teachers of Oral Pathology. Oral Surg Oral Med Oral Pathol Oral Radiol Endod. 1997;83:672–9.

Beacher NG, Brodie MJ, Goodall C. A case report: retigabine induced oral mucosal dyspigmentation of the hard palate. BMC Oral Health. 2015;15:122.

Buchner A, Hansen LS. Pigmented nevi of the oral mucosa: a clinico pathologic study of 36 new cases and review of 155 cases from the literature. Part II: analysis of 191 cases. Oral Surg Oral Med Oral Pathol Oral Radiol Endod. 1987;63:676–82.

Eisen D. Disorders of pigmentation in the oral cavity. Clin Dermatol. 2000;18:579–87.

Goode RK, Crawford BE, Callihan MD, Neville BW. Oral melanoacanthoma. Review of the literature and report of ten cases. Oral Surg Oral Med Oral Pathol Oral Radiol Endod. 1983;56(6):622–8.

Hedin CA, Pindborg JJ, Daftary DK, Mehta FS. Melanin depigmentation of the palatal mucosa in reverse smokers: a preliminary study. J Oral Pathol Med. 1992;21:440–4.

Hemminki A. The molecular basis and clinical aspects of Peutz-Jeghers syndrome. Cell Mol Life Sci. 1999;55(5):735–50.

Hicks MJ, Flaitz CM. Oral mucosal melanoma: epidemiology and pathobiology. Oral Oncol. 2000;36(2):152–69.

Hussaini HM, Waddell JN, West LM, et al. Silver solder « tattoo » a novel form of oral pigmentation identified with the use of field emission electron microscopy and electron dispersive spectrography. Oral Surg Oral Med Oral Pathol Oral Radiol Endod. 2011;112:6–10.

Joska L, Venclikova Z, Poddana M, Berada O. The mechanism of gingival metallic pigmentation formation. Clin Oral Investig. 2009;13(1):1–7.

Kauzman A, Pavone M, Blanas N, Bradley G. Pigmented lesions of the oral cavity: review, differential diagnosis, and case presentations. J Can Dent Assoc. 2004;70(10):682–3.

Kleinegger CL, Hammond HL, Finkelstein MW. Oral mucosal hyperpigmentation secondary to antimalarial drug therapy. Oral Surg Oral Med Oral Pathol Oral Radiol Endod. 2000;90:189–94.

Li CC, Malik SM, Blaeser BF, et al. Mucosal pigmentation caused by imatinib: report of three cases. Head Neck Pathol. 2012;6:290–5.

Lyne A, Creedon A, Bailey BMN. Mucosal pigmentation of the hard palate in a patient taking imatinib. BMJ Case Rep. 2015;2015:1–13. https://doi.org/10.1136/bcr-2015-209335.

Meleti M, Vescovi P, Mooi WJ, van der Waal I. Pigmented lesions of the oral mucosa and perioral tissues: a flowchart for the diagnosis and some recommendations for the management. Oral Surg Oral Med Oral Pathol Oral Radiol Endod. 2008;105(5):606–16.

Mergoni G, Ergun S, Vescovi P, et al. Oral postinflammatory pigmentation: an analysis of 7 cases. Med Oral Patol Oral Cir Bucal. 2011;16(1):e11–4.

Nikitakis NG, Koumaki D. Laugier-Hunziger syndrome: case report and review of the literature. Oral Surg Oral Med Oral Pathol Oral Radiol Endod. 2013;116(1):e52–8.

Pichard DC, Boyee AM, Collins MT, Lowen EW. Oral pigmentation in McCune-Albright syndrome. JAMA Dermatol. 2014;150(7):760–3.

Sarkar SB, Sarkar S, Ghosh S, Bandyopadhyay S. Addison's disease. Contemp Clin Dent. 2012;3(4):484–6.

Shkolnik TG, Feuerman H, Didkovsky E, et al. Blue-gray mucocutaneous discoloration: a new adverse effect of exogabine. JAMA Dermatol. 2014;150(9):984–9.

Turakji B, Umair A, Prasad D, Altamini MA. Diagnosis of oral pigmentations and malignant transformations. Singapore Dent J. 2014;35:39–46.

Vera-Sirena B, Risueno-Mata P, Ricart-Vaya JM, Ruiz de la Hermosa CB, Vera-Sempere F. Clinicopathological and immunohistochemical study of oral amalgam pigmentation. Acta Otorinolaringol Esp. 2012;63(5):376–81.

Westbury IW, Najera A. Minocycline-induced intraoral pharmacogenic pigmentation: case reports and review of the literature. J Periodontol. 1997;68:84–91.

Yarom N, Epstein J, Levi H, et al. Oral manifestations of habitual khat chewing: a case-control study. Oral Surg Oral Med Oral Pathol Oral Radiol Endod. 2010;109:60–6.

Zaraa I, Labbene I, El Guellali N, et al. Kaposi's sarcoma: epidemiological, clinical, anatomopathological and therapeutic features in 75 patients. Tunis Med. 2012;90(2):116–21.

Drug-Induced Oral Ulcers

Sara Laurencin-Dalicieux and Sarah Cousty

1 General Considerations

Ulceration is characterized by a more or less profound loss of substance of the surface epithelium and exposing the underlying chorion.

Ulcerations of the oral mucosa are a frequent cause of consultation, as pain induced by this lesion is a frequent functional sign. The etiologies of oral ulcerations are multiple: trauma, deficiency diseases, infectious, hematological, malignant, etc. (Fig. 1, Table 1).

Some are induced by drug medications. The exact diagnosis may be difficult.

The most well-known drug-induced oral ulcerations are those induced by chemotherapy,

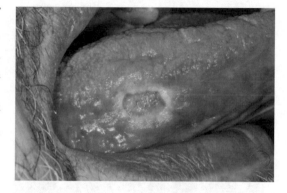

Fig. 1 Chronic traumatic ulceration in a diabetic patient

S. Laurencin-Dalicieux (✉)
Periodontology Department, Dental Faculty, Paul Sabatier University, Toulouse, France

Periodontology Department, CHU de Toulouse, Toulouse, France

CERPOP, UMR INSERM 1295, Paul Sabatier University, Toulouse, France
e-mail: laurencin.s@chu-toulouse.fr

S. Cousty
Oral Surgery Oral Medecine Department, Dental Faculty, Paul Sabatier University, Toulouse, France

Oral Surgery Oral Medecine Department, CHU de Toulouse, Toulouse, France

LAPLACE, UMR CNRS 5213, Paul Sabatier University, Toulouse, France
e-mail: cousty.s@chu-toulouse.fr

associated with an important acute pain that often requires cessation of chemotherapy. In the oral mucosa, drug-induced oral ulceration can be secondary infected by opportunistic organisms (fungi, bacteria), especially in the case of an immune-depressive treatment.

Many others etiologies should be noted:

- Some ulcerations may be due to direct trauma: it is a misuse of the drug (Figs. 2 and 3).
- Some ulcerations may be due to deficiencies induced by long-term medication use (Table 2). It is well known that there is a significant association of deficiencies of hemoglobin, iron, vitamin B12, ferritin, and folic acid levels with recurrent aphthous stomatitis (Fig. 4). As a result, any medication that may induce these deficits is likely to indirectly induce multiple oral ulcerations.

© Springer Nature Switzerland AG 2021
S. Cousty, S. Laurencin-Dalicieux (eds.), *Drug-Induced Oral Complications*,
https://doi.org/10.1007/978-3-030-66973-7_4

Table 1 Major diagnoses of oral ulcerations (excluding drug-induced oral ulcers)

Single ulceration	Multiple ulcerations	Recurrent ulcerations
Acute Aphtosis (Fig. 4) Traumatic ulcer Eosinophilic ulcer	*Acute* Aphtosis military Post-bullous and post-vesicular ulcers Necrotizing ulcerative gingivitis	Aphtosis Behcet's disease Cyclic neutropenia Infectious ulcers (herpes viruses, HIV, …) Neutrophilic dermatosis Chronic inflammatory bowel disease (IDB) Deficiency disease ulcerations Eosinophilic ulcer
Chronic Malignant tumor Infectious ulceration (syphilis) Necrotizing sialometaplasia Autoimmune disease (arteritis) Traumatic ulcer (Fig. 1)	*Chronic* Hematologic diseases (leukemia, …) Autoimmune diseases Chronic inflammatory bowel disease (IDB)	

Table 2 Medicinal products known to be associated with deficiencies

Proton pump inhibitors	Iron deficiency
Isotretinoin	Vitamin B12 deficiency
Histamine-2 receptor antagonists	Ferritin deficiency

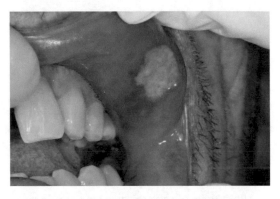

Fig. 4 Aphthous ulceration (52-year-old man)

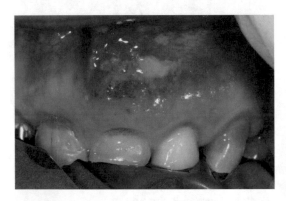

Fig. 2 Traumatic ulceration due to direct application of effervescent tablet

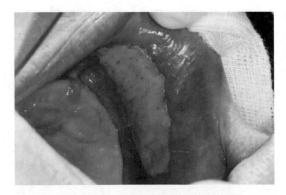

Fig. 3 Traumatic ulceration due to direct application of essential oils

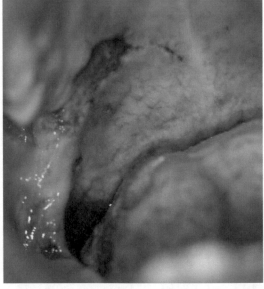

Fig. 5 Post-bullous ulceration (pemphigus in a 17-year-old patient)

Oral ulcerations may appear immediately or may result from bubbles or vesicles. Post-bullous ulcerations are rarer in drug etiology (Fig. 5). They may appear in the context of drug-induced toxidermia or autoimmune bullous diseases induced by medications. The pathophysiological mechanisms leading to drug-induced oral ulcers remain unclear.

2 Aphthous-Like and Non-aphtous-Like Ulcers

These ulcerations are often considered as chronic ulcers; they last for 2 weeks or longer. They can be solitary or multiple. The drugs responsible for the lesions are various (Table 3).

2.1 NSAIDs

These drugs were one of the earliest classes of molecules associated with aphthous-like ulcers in the oral cavity. In particular, piroxicam was incriminated, possibly because of its thiol group.

Naproxen and cyclooxygenase-2 inhibitors (e.g., rofecoxib) can also induce oral ulcerations.

2.2 Nicorandil (Fig. 6)

It is a nicotinamide ester and a potassium channel activator used in the prevention and long-term treatment of angina pectoris. This drug has been first used in Japan. It was introduced in Europe over 20 years ago.

Table 3 Table of principal medications causing oral ulcerations

NSAIDs	Piroxicam, Naproxen, Indometacin, cyclooxygenase-2 inhibitors
Cardiology	Anti-anginal agent (nicorandil) Antihypertensive agent, angiotensin receptor blocker (sartan) Antiplatelet drugs
Immunosuppressant	Tacrolimus, sirolimus, temsirolimus, everolimus, ridaforolimus, and mycophenolate mofetil
Anticancer agent	mTorr, conventional chemotherapy agents, MTKIs
Psychiatry	Antidepressants, neuroleptics, thymoregulators

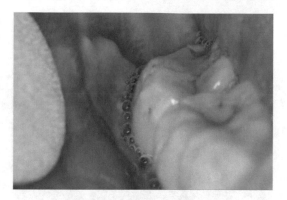

Fig. 6 Nicorandil-induced ulceration in a 45-year-old woman

Ulcerations due to Nicorandil can be located on the mucosa (oral, anal, and digestive mucosa), and also on the skin. Tongue ulcerations are the most frequent. Oral ulcerations can be unique or multiple. Their size ranges from 1 to 3 cm. Unlike aphtosis, there is no erythematous halo.

2.3 Immunosuppressant (Fig. 7) (Tacrolimus, Sirolimus, Temsirolimus, Everolimus, Ridaforolimus, and Mycophenolate Mofetil)

On cessation of these medications, these ulcerations regress completely without recurrence. These molecules can also promote the development of opportunistic infections with mucous manifestation such as herpes.

Conventional Chemotherapy Agents (Fig. 8) (5-Fluorouracil, Cisplatin, Methotrexate, Hydroxyurea)

Ulcers are usually large and diffuse in the oral mucosa.

Direct toxicity or toxicity mediated by immunosuppressive effect might be the mechanisms of inducing oral ulcerations.

Severe neutropenia is a well-known cause of oral ulceration. Neutropenia is defined as an ANC of <1500 cells/mm^3 for most adults and children. Neutropenia can be graded as mild, moderate, and severe, corresponding respectively to ANC values of 1000–1500, 500–1000, and <500 cells/mm^3.

The most common cause of acutely acquired neutropenia is cytotoxic chemotherapy for malig-

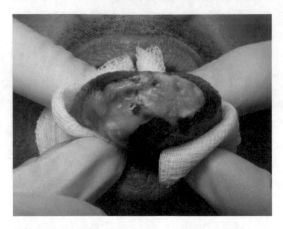

Fig. 7 Tacrolimus-induced ulceration in a renal transplanted patient

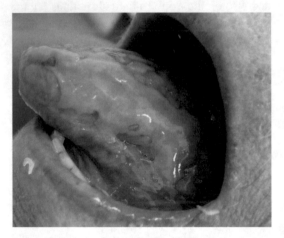

Fig. 8 Ulceration-induced by chemotherapy. (Courtesy Dr. Chaux-Bodard Anne Gaëlle)

Table 4 Principal causes of drug-induced neutropenia

Direct marrow suppression	Chloramphenicol and phenothiazines
Immune destruction of the neutrophil or myeloid precursors	Penicillins, cephalosporins, and quinidine

nant diseases (20–40% of patients given chemotherapy). It can be induced by medications (Table 4).

Other drugs, such as anticholinergics, bronchodilators, vasodilators, allopurinol, have been reported to induce oral ulcerations. However, their causality assessment remains difficult to prove.

3 Bullous Disorders

They can be considered as acute ulcers. Most of the time, they are multiple ulcerative lesions. They can be autoimmune or not. Diagnosis is based on clinical examination, anatomopathological, and immunohistochemical examination. Bullous lesions quickly give way to more or less deep ulcerations, due to repeated microtrauma: mastication, phonation, etc.

3.1 Medication-Induced Autoimmune Bullous Disorders

They are rare in oral mucosa and causality assessment remains unclear.

3.1.1 Pemphigus
(Fig. 9: Multiple ulcerations in pemphigus)

Bullous lesions are suprabasal and intraepidermal. Epidermal cells lose their cohesion (acantholysis). The main drugs responsible of such lesions are the thiol radical-containing drugs such as penicillin and NSAIDs (Table 5).

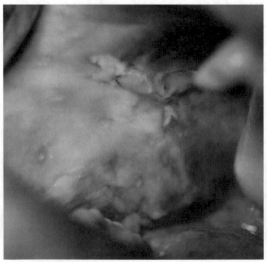

Fig. 9 Multiple ulcerations in pemphigus

Table 5 Principal causes of drug-induced pemphigus

Cardiology	Angiotensin-converting enzyme inhibitors Calcium channels blockers Captopril, nifedipine
NSAIDs	Diclofenac, piroxicam
Antibiotic	Penicillin, rifampicin

3.1.2 Bullous Pemphigoid

(Fig. 10: Ulceration in mucous membrane pemphigoid)

Bullous lesions involve the subepidermal basal lamina area. During the last decade, an increased prevalence of diabetes mellitus in bullous pemphigoid patients has been observed. It could be linked with the dipeptidyl peptidase-4 inhibitor, which can be prescribed in the treatment of type 2 diabetes mellitus (Table 6).

3.1.3 Lupus Erythematosus and Bullous LEB

It is a very rare clinical presentation of systemic lupus erythematosus. Some drugs can be related with LEB: procainamide, hydralazine, and biologic agents (anti-TNF inhibitors).

3.1.4 Linear IgA Dermatosis

It is an autoimmune disease that may be drug-induced. It is characterized by blisters with a tense clinical appearance due to linear deposition of IgA and disruption of the dermo–epidermal junction. The main offending drug is an antibiotic: vancomycin (Table 7).

3.2 Medication-Induced Non-autoimmune Bullous Disorders

3.2.1 Erythema Multiforme (EM): Major or Minor

EM is an acute reaction that affects both the skin and mucous membranes (Figs. 11, 12, and 13).It is most commonly linked to an infectious agent, such as herpes simplex virus and less commonly to mycoplasma pneumonia (especially in children). It is a hypersensitivity reaction. Approximately

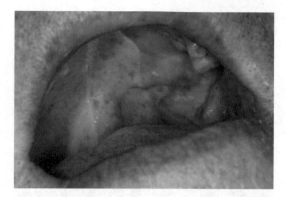

Fig. 10 Ulceration in mucous membrane pemphigoid

Table 6 Principal causes of drug-induced pemphigoid

Cardiology	Angiotensin-converting enzyme inhibitors Beta-blockers Diuretics
NSAIDs	Diclofenac, piroxicam, ibuprofen
Antibiotic	Penicillin, cephalosporine, rifampicin, quinolone
Hypoglycemic (type 2 diabetes mellitus)	Dipeptidyl peptidase-4 inhibitor (to be confirmed)

Table 7 Principal causes of drug-induced linear IgA dermatosis

Cardiology	Captopril, verapamil, atorvastatin, furosemide, amiodarone
NSAIDs	Diclofenac, piroxicam, naproxen
Antibiotic	Penicillin, cephalosporin, vancomycin
Anticonvulsant	Phenytoin, carbamazepine

18% of the cases present hypersensitivity reactions to medications (Table 8).

Clinically, it presents as irregular oral ulcers with diffuse erythema. Target-shaped lesions should also be searched for on the skin.

3.2.2 Steven Johnson Syndrome (SJS) and Toxic Epidermal Necrolysis (TEN) (Fig. 14)

They are severe necrolytic hypersensitivity reactions. Unlike EM, they are much more frequently associated with the use of medications. They can be life-threatening. In TEN, more than 30% of

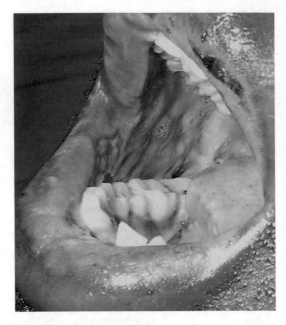

Fig. 11 Erythema multiforme

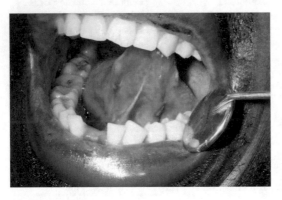

Fig. 12 Erythema multiforme

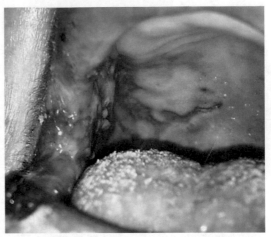

Fig. 13 Erythema multiforme

Table 8 Major medications implicated in EM

NSAI
Antimicrobials (amoxicillin/clavulanic acid, cephalosporin, tetracycline, macrolide, sulfonamides)
Anticonvulsants (phenytoin)
Monoclonal antibodies (infliximab and adalimumab)

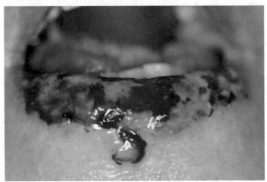

Fig. 14 Steven Johnson syndrome

Table 9 Major medications implicated in TEN

Antimicrobials (amoxicillin/clavulanic acid)
Anticonvulsants (phenytoin, lamotrigine)
Allopurinol
Rituximab
NSAI
Nevirapine
Carbamazepine
Sulfonamide

the mucosal skin surface is affected, and about one-third of the patients die.

In SJS and TEN, the mucous membranes of the mouth, eye, and genitalia are involved. Different medications have been implicated (Table 9).

3.2.3 DRESS Syndrome: Drug Rash with Eosinophilia and Systemic Symptoms Syndrome

This is a drug hypersensitivity reaction. Clinical presentation sometimes mimics a toxic epidermal necrolysis reaction. Mucosal and skin lesions appear from 6 to 8 weeks after the beginning of the drug administration (Table 10).

Table 10 Major medications implicated in DRESS syndrome

Anticonvulsants
Allopurinol
Sulfonamide
Cyclosporine
Azathioprine

4   Conclusion

Oral ulcerations are common in the pathology of oral mucosa. They may be due to a drug, especially when they are chronic, persistent, or recurrent. The accountability of a drug is often difficult to establish. Many differential diagnoses need to be discussed. The diagnosis of squamous cell carcinoma should not be forgotten.

Bibliography

Asare K, Gatzke CB. Mycophenolate-inducedoral ulcers: case report and literature review. Am J Health Syst Pharm. 2020;77(7):523–8.

Balakumar P, Kavitha M, Suresh Nanditha S. Cardiovascular drugs-induced oral toxicities: a murky area to be revisited and illuminated. Pharmacol Res. 2015;102:81–9.

Boulinguez S, Reix S, Bedane C, Debrock C, Bouyssou-Gauthier ML, Sparsa A, et al. Role of drug exposure in aphtous ulcers: a case-control study. Br J Dermatol. 2000;143:1261–5.

Fania L, Di Zenzo G, Didona B, Pilla MA, Sobrino L, Panebianco A, Mazzanti C, Abeni D. Increased prevalence of diabetes mellitus in bullous pemphigoid patients during the last decade. J Eur Acad Dermatol Venereol. 2018;32(4):e153–4.

Liabeuf S, Gras V, Moragny J, Laroche ML, Andrejak M. Ulceration of the mucosa following direct contact with ferrous sulfate in eldery patients: a case report and a review of the French national pharmacovigilance database. Clin Interv Aging. 2014;9:737–40.

Ozkaya E. Oral mucosal fixed drug eruption: characteristics and differential diagnosis. J Am Acad Dermatol. 2013;69:e51–8.

Philipone E, Rockafellow A, Sternberg R, Yoon A, Koslovsky D. Oral ulcerations as a sequela of tacrolimus and mycophenolate mofetil therapy. Oral Surg Oral Med Oral Pathol Oral Radiol. 2014;118:e175–8.

Scully C, Bagan JV. Adverse drug reactions in the orofacial region. Crit Rev Oral Biol Med. 2004;15:221–39.

Yuan A, Woo SB. Adverse drug events in the oral cavity. Oral Surg Oral Med Oral Pathol Oral Radiol. 2015;119:35–47.

Drug-Induced Oral Lichenoid Reaction

Jean-Christophe Fricain

1 Definition

Idiopathic lichen planus is an inflammatory disease characterized clinically by cutaneous papules and a keratinized network crosslinked at the level of the oral mucosa.

The typical histological aspect is an inflammatory lympho-plasmocytic infiltrate under the basal membrane responsible for the formation of apoptotic bodies.

Some drugs or local trauma can induce clinically and histologically lichenoid lesions of oral lichen planus. However, these lesions generally regress with suppression of the cause which distinguish them from true lesions of oral lichen planus.

Lichen planus and lichenoïd lesions can be observed on skin and mucosa. Oral and genital mucosa are the main localizations.

2 Epidemiology

The prevalence of drug-induced lichenoid reactions is poorly understood and probably underestimated due to diagnostic difficulties and the prospective of studies.

J.-C. Fricain (✉)
Inserm U1026 "Bioingénierie Tissulaire – BioTis",
UFR d'odontologie, Université Bordeaux,
Bordeaux Cedex, France
e-mail: jean-christophe.fricain@inserm.fr

In the PubMed database, less than 300 articles have reported a cutaneous or oral lichenoid reaction and only half have exploitable imputability criteria. 42.2% of patients had strict cutaneous manifestations, 20% of patients had strict mucosal manifestations, and 26% of patients showed cutaneous and mucosal manifestations. In 131 patients, the delay between drug intake and onset of lichenoid reaction was 155 days with a minimum of 2 h and a maximum of 6 years.

The majority of drug-induced lichenoid reactions published in the literature are case reports. The mean age of lichenoid reactions varies from 44 to 66 years depending on onset of pathologies for which inducer drugs are prescribed.

3 Inductive Drugs

The most accountable and most frequently cited treatments are penicillamines and gold salts (sodium aurothiopropanolsulfonate) but they are not really used nowadays.

To a lesser extent, most frequently cited treatments are:

- ACE inhibitors (captopril, ramipril, enalapril).
- Beta blockers (propranolol, sotalol, labetalol).
- Tyrosine kinase inhibitor targeting BCR-AB (imatinib).

Other drugs have been associated more rarely with the onset of a lichenoid reaction. Among others:

- Non-steroidal anti-inflammatory drugs (indomethacin).
- Diuretics (hydrochlorothiazide).
- Hypoglycemic sulfonamides.
- Immunomodulators (sulfasalazine).
- Antiparkinsonian (methyldopa).
- Anti-epileptics (carbamazepine).
- Antiretrovirals (protease inhibitors).
- Cholesterol-lowering agents (simvastatin, pravastatin).
- Treatments for gout (allopurinol).

Interestingly, drugs sometimes used to treat lichen planus can also induce lichenoid reactions: dapsone, levamisole, tetracyclines, and IFN-α.

It should also be pointed out that literature is enriched with new observations with some innovative treatments such as: anti-TNFα (Tumor necrosis factor α) used in rheumatology (rheumatoid arthritis), dermatology (psoriasis), or gastroenterology (Crohn's disease): infliximab, adalimumab; immunological checkpoint inhibitors targeting PD-1 or PD-L1 used in oncology: nivolumab, pembrolizumab, atezolizumab.

4 Physiopathology

4.1 The Pathophysiology of Lichenoid Reactions of Drug Origin Is Not Well Known

As for the LP, lichenoid reactions are due to an autoimmune mechanism induced by T lymphocytes that attack epidermal cells. Breathnach et al. believe that lichenoid reactions may be due to self-reactive cytotoxic T lymphocyte clones directed against drug antigens such that keratinocytes and Langerhans cells are perceived as non-self. Shiohara et al. report a correlation between the presence of epidermotropic cytotoxic T lymphocytes in lichenoid reactions in mice after an injection.

It seems that the mechanism depends on the drug used.

For penicillamines, it is known that this family of medicinal products leads to a modification of the cell surface antigens which may explain the immune reaction leading to a lichenoid reaction.

For anti-inflammatory drugs like naproxen, inhibition of cyclo-oxygenase could lead to lichenoid reaction.

The occurrence of lichenoid reactions under beta-blocker may also suggest an adrenergic mechanism.

Some drugs—penicillamines, some converting enzyme (captopril) inhibitors, and gold salts—have a common thiol group that could participate in the immune reaction.

A polymorphism of the enzymes of the cytochrome P450, at the origin of a deficiency of hepatic metabolism of the drugs, can also participate in this mucous toxicity.

Concerning the anti-TNFα, the evoked mechanism is an overproduction of interferon alpha which activates the dendritic cells and the T lymphocytes.

5 Histology

The dermo–epidermal junction is the site of lichenoid reactions. The histological examination of a cutaneous-mucosal lesion is a major argument in the establishment of a diagnosis. 82.2% of the reported cases have histology consistent with the lichenoid reaction. Compared histologically to the lichen planus, lichenoid reactions are distinguished by the worst limitation of the infiltrate, which is also less monomorphic, and may include eosinophilic or neutrophilic polynuclear cells and plasma cells. However, it is very difficult to distinguish lichen planus from lichenoid reaction. Other pathologies such as erythema multiforme, lupus erythematosus, dermatomyositis, and GVH are histologically close to the drug-induced lichenoid reactions, but the clinical picture makes it possible to rule out these diagnoses.

6 Positive Diagnosis

Usually, drug-induced lichenoid reaction is evoked in the context of the introduction of a new treatment. The duration of onset of lichenoid lesions varies widely, ranging from 2 weeks to a few months.

The diagnosis of drug-induced lichenoid reaction is based on two points:

1. *The clinical and para-clinical diagnosis of a lichenoid lesion.*

   The clinical criteria most often proposed are oral lichenoid lesions that remain unilateral, with an erosive aspect. However, these criteria are not specific because medicated lichenoid reactions can develop bilaterally and be plurifocal. Moreover, it is likely that the diagnosis is more often made at the erosive stage, more painful, than at the keratosic stage.

   In practice, these lichenoid reactions can be described as four elementary lesions: erythema (Fig. 1), erosion (Fig. 2), ulceration (Fig. 3), and keratosis (Fig. 4), the latter often assuming a striated or fern leaf-like appearance.

   Histopathological examination, although often not specific and comparable to idiopathic lichen planus, can sometimes lead to a medicinal origin by the presence of a more diffuse inflammatory infiltrate, with polynuclear eosinophils and numerous apoptotic bodies.

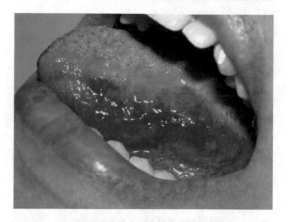

Fig. 2 Interferon-induced oral lichenoid reaction dominated by erosions

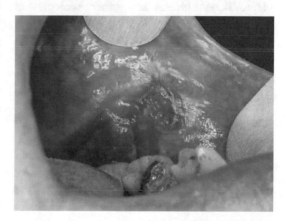

Fig. 3 Allopurinol-induced oral lichenoid ulcer

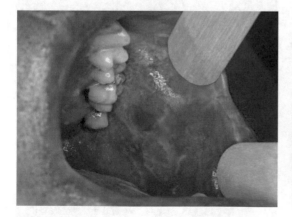

Fig. 1 Indomethacin-induced oral lichenoid reaction dominated by erythematous aspect

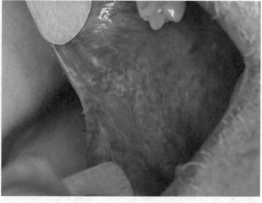

Fig. 4 Naproxen-induced oral lichenoid reaction dominated by keratosis

2. *Its drug imputability.*

Diagnosis of drug-induced oral lichenoïd reaction is based on imputability criteria. There are many methods for evaluating imputability, but the main criteria are: time to appear after the drug has been introduced, relapse after treatment discontinuation, absence or associated treatment, a known pharmacological mechanism, and recurrence after reintroduction of the drug.

7 Differencial Diagnosis

The main differential diagnoses include idiopathic lichen planus and other etiologies of lichenoid reactions.

7.1 Idiopathic Oral Lichen Planus

The idiopathic oral lichen planus represents 20% of the consultations of oral mucosa diseases. Its prevalence in the general adult population is estimated to be between 0.5 and 2%.

Oral lichen planus is a chronic, progressive disease. The keratinized lesions often evolve from a dotted stage (Fig. 5) which becomes crosslinked (Fig. 6) and then into a plaque (Fig. 7) which sometimes assumes a verrucous appearance (Fig. 8). The transition from a purely keratosic form to an erythematous (Fig. 9), erosive (Fig. 10), or ulcerated (Fig. 11) form is common.

Stress could be a factor of evolution. Lichen planus should be considered as a potentially malignant lesion. Approximately 1–3% of chronic lesions of oral lichen are likely to degenerate into squamous cell carcinoma (Fig. 12).

The differential diagnosis with drug-induced oral lichenoid lesions is mainly based on imputability criteria because lesions are very similar from both clinical and histological points of view.

The diagnosis of drug-induced lichenoid reaction should be evoke when lesions appear during the introduction of a new drug or when a patient takes a treatment known to induce

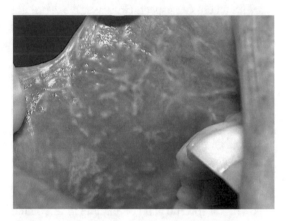

Fig. 6 Oral lichen planus with crosslinked keratosis

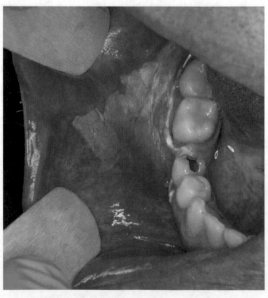

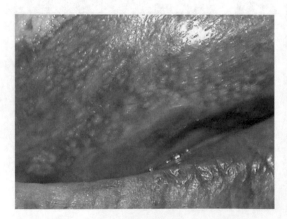

Fig. 5 Oral lichen planus at dotted stage

Fig. 7 Plaque of oral lichen planus

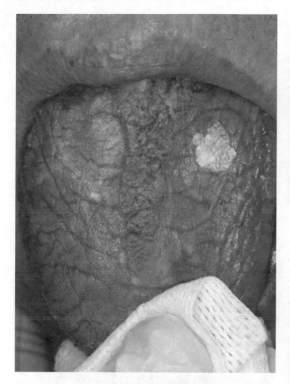

Fig. 8 Verrucous aspect of oral lichen planus

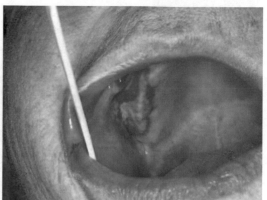

Fig. 10 Erosive oral lichen planus

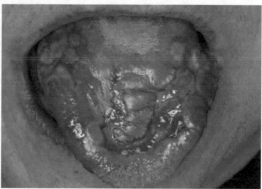

Fig. 11 Ulcerative oral lichen planus

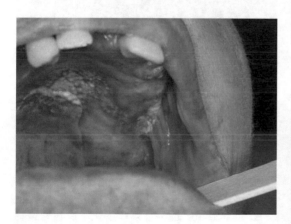

Fig. 9 Erythematous and keratosis oral lichen planus

lichenoid reactions and the lesions of lichen do not have a usual course.

7.2 Contact Lichenoid Lesions

They generally result from a Koebner phenomenon, that is to say from the development of a lichen-

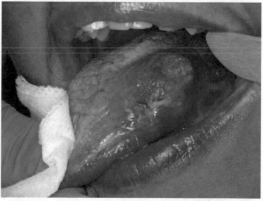

Fig. 12 Squamous cell carcinoma developed on oral lichen planus

oid lesion on an area which has undergone repeated microtrauma. These lichenoid contact lesions must be evoked before lesions are limited to certain spe-

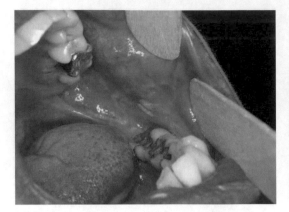

Fig. 13 Contact lichenoid reaction

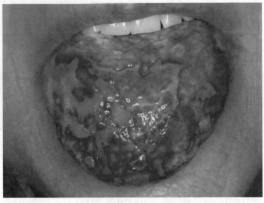

Fig. 14 Oral lichenoid reaction in GVH

cific buccal areas. For example, they are particularly frequent in the jugular mucosa, in relation to the molars, especially if they are in malposition, amalgamated, or crowned (Fig. 13). The replacement of fillings, prosthetic crowns, or the avulsion of the teeth generally allows the disappearance of these lichenoid reactions. On the other hand, if the lesions are related to a limited idiopathic lichen planus, these dental treatments remain ineffective and the diagnosis must be reconsidered.

Few authors have incriminated a mechanism of contact hypersensitivity but this remains unclear. In practice, the removal of amalgams can be proposed in case of strong suspicion but we will refrain from modifying the prostheses in the majority of cases.

7.3 Lichenoid Lesion of Graft Versus Host Disease

Lichenoid lesions may occur as a result of an allogeneic bone marrow transplant as part of a graft-versus-host reaction (aggression of the recipient's skin or mucosal antigens by donor lymphocytes).

These lesions have a high clinical similarity with idiopathic lichen planus but are often more extensive and more inflammatory (Fig. 14). They require regular follow-up because there is a risk of degeneration in immunocompromised patients. The clinical context of the lesions and their severity allows the differential diagnoses with drug-induced lichenoid reaction.

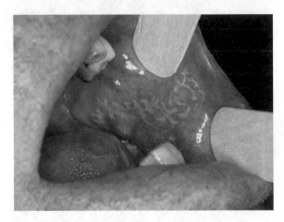

Fig. 15 Lichenoid lesion associated with hepatitis C

7.4 Lichenoid Lesions Associated with General Disease

- Hepatitis C: Oral lichenoid lesions have frequently been reported in countries where hepatitis C is endemic. In this context, it is important to search for hepatitis C when a lichenoid lesion is observed (Fig. 15). Hepatitis C is sometimes treated with Interferon gamma which can induce lichenoid lesion. In this case, the diagnosis is usually made a posteriori when lesion relapses after treatment cessation.

- APECED: Oral lichenoid lesions have been reported in APECED syndrome (autoimmune polyendocrinopathy-candidiasis-ectodermal dystrophy). This exceptional disease is autosomal recessive and is characterized by the association of autoimmune endocrine involvement, cutaneous-mucosal candidiasis and ectodermal

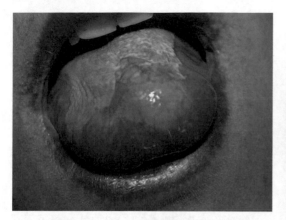

Fig. 16 Lichenoid lesion in APECED syndrome

tissue damage. They would result from the absence of destruction of the self-reactive T lymphocytes by mutation of the AIRE gene. The frequent progression of lichenoid lesions to epidermoid carcinoma in the APECED syndrome requires regular monitoring. The differential diagnostic with drug-induced lichenoid reaction is easy due to clinical context (Fig. 16).

- Good syndrome: Oral lichenoid lesions have been described several times in Good syndrome (Fig. 17). It manifests by a thymoma associated with hypogammaglobulinemia, circulating B lymphopenia, circulating CD4 T lymphopenia with an inverted CD4/CD8 ratio. It is complicated by infections and autoimmune diseases such as lichenoid lesions. The differential diagnosis with drug-induced lichenoid reaction is easily done due to clinical context.

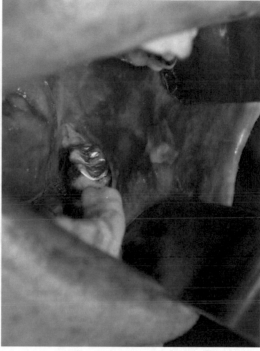

Fig. 17 Lichenoid lesion in Good syndrome

required and a biopsy is not systematic. A simple annual monitoring is required.

- Atypical keratosis, thick, inhomogeneous, more or less indurated: a biopsy is necessary. If it reveals a lichenoid lesion, it will be necessary to look for a medicinal cause. Due to the suspicious nature, drug withdrawal will be advocated according to its indication and the possibilities of substitution.
- Keratosis typical of lichen and multiple ulcerations, flexible on palpation: a treatment with local corticotherapy (clobetasol in particular) is established. If the lesions remain inflammatory, a biopsy is required and the medical examination must seek a medicinal cause. If a drug is suspected, its withdrawal is recommended based on its indication and possible substitution.
- Typical lichen keratosis with or without ulceration appeared after introduction of treatment: a suspicion of lichenoid lesion can be made immediately and an eviction will be advocated according to its indication and the possibilities of substitution.

8   Treatment

Treatment of drug-induced lichenoid lesions is based on drug withdrawal. The regression of the lesion will occur several weeks or months after.

In general, the diagnosis of drug-induced lichenoid is evoked in second intention. In all cases, local corticosteroids are instituted but depending on the appearance and the evolution of the lesions, different attitudes are possible:

- Keratosis with typical aspect of lichen, not painful, flexible on palpation: no treatment is

Bibliography

Bonerandi JJ. Le patron lichénoïde: Expression histologique des agressions de l'interface dermo-épidermique. Rev Médecine Interne. 2003;24:9s–11s.

Breathnach S. Mechanisms of drug eruptions: part I. Australas J Dermatol. 1995;36(3):121–7.

Campana F, Fricain JC, Sibaud V, Vigarios E. Toxicité buccale des médicaments. Malakoff: Ed CDP; 2016. p. 197.

Chugh S, Sarkar R, Garg VK, Singh A, Keisham C. Multifocal fixed drug eruption with COX-2 inhibitor-celecoxib. Indian J Dermatol. 2013;58(2):142–4.

Cortés-Ramírez DA, Rodríguez-Tojo MJ, Gainza-Cirauqui ML, Martínez-Conde R, Aguirre-Urizar JM. Overexpression of cyclooxygenase-2 as a biomarker in different subtypes of the oral lichenoid disease. Oral Surg Oral Med Oral Pathol Oral Radiol Endodontol. 2010;110(6):738–43.

Halevy S, Shai A. Lichenoid drug eruptions. J Am Acad Dermatol. 1993;29(2 Part 1):249–55.

Heymann WR, Lerman JS, Luftschein S. Naproxen-induced lichen planus. J Am Acad Dermatol. 1984;10(2 Pt 1):299–301.

Kamath VV, Setlur K, Yerlagudda K. Oral lichenoid lesions—a review and update. Indian J Dermatol. 2015;60(1):102.

Krupaa RJ, Sankari SL, Masthan KMK, Rajesh E. Oral lichen planus: an overview. J Pharm Bioallied Sci. 2015;7(Suppl 1):S158–61.

Lage D, Juliano PB, Metze K, de Souza EM, Cintra ML. Lichen planus and lichenoid drug-induced eruption: a histological and immunohistochemical study. Int J Dermatol. 2012;51(10):1199–205.

Lukács J, Schliemann S, Elsner P. Lichen planus and lichenoid reactions as a systemic disease. Clin Dermatol. 2015;33(5):512–9.

Macedo AF, Marques FB, Ribeiro CF, Teixeira F. Causality assessment of adverse drug reaction: comparison of the results obtained from publish decisional algorithms and from the evaluations of an expert panel, according to different levels of imputability. J Clin Pharm Ther. 2003;28(2):137–43.

Shiohara T, Mizukawa Y. The immunological basis of lichenoid tissue reaction. Autoimmun Rev. 2005;4(4):236–41.

Shiohara T, Moriya N, Nagashima M. The lichenoid tissue reaction. Int J Dermatol. 1988;27(6):365–74.

Medication-Related Osteonecrosis of the Jaws

Leonor Costa Mendes and Bruno Courtois

1 Introduction

Osteonecrosis of the jaws induced by drugs, also called osteochemonecrosis, is defined as an area of exposed bone in the maxilla or mandible that does not heal over a period of 6–8 weeks. It is a well-known side effect of bisphosphonate therapy, first described by Marx in 2003. More recently, osteonecrosis of the jaws (ONJ) was observed as an undesirable effect of other drugs, such as denosumab (a monoclonal antibody with inhibition power of osteoclastic activity) and other antiangiogenic cancer therapies.

2 Inducting Drugs

2.1 Osteoclastic Activity Inhibitors

2.1.1 Bisphosphonates

Bisphosphonates (BP) are structural analogs of inorganic pyrophosphate presenting a high affinity for hydroxyapatite crystals, especially on bony surfaces undergoing active resorption. They are powerful inhibitors of osteoclastic function and differentiation and increase osteoclastic apoptosis, thus preventing bone remodeling. BPs are used to treat osteoporosis, several metabolic bone diseases (Paget's disease, osteogenesis imperfecta, osteopenia), and cancer-related conditions such as bone metastases from solid tumors or lytic lesions caused by multiple myeloma.

BPs can be divided into two classes: non-aminobisphosphonates, or first-generation BPs, and aminobisphosphonates (NBPs), comprising second- and third-generation BPs. NBPs have much higher inhibition potency in comparison to first-generation BPs; this is due to the presence of a nitrogen group in the molecule's long side chain. First-generation bisphosphonates include etidronate, clodronate, and tiludronate. Second-generation bisphosphonates are pamidronate and alendronate, and third-generation BPs comprise risedronate, ibandronate, and zoledronic acid, the most powerful antiresorptive molecule.

Bisphosphonates present a low intestinal absorption: intravenous administration is thereby favored in oncologic treatments. These drugs are also resistant to enzymatic and chemical breakdown, which means they can be incorporated into the skeleton without being degraded, making them remarkably persistent drugs; the estimated half-life of alendronate can attain 12 years.

2.1.2 RANK-L Inhibitors: Denosumab

Osteoclast activity is regulated by RANK/RANK-L/OPG signaling (RANK: receptor activator of nuclear factor-κB; RANKL: RANK ligand; OPG: osteoprotegerin). An increase in RANK-L

L. Costa Mendes · B. Courtois (✉)
Dental faculty, Paul Sabatier University, Toulouse, France

Oral surgery Oral Medicine Department, CHU Toulouse, Toulouse, France

© Springer Nature Switzerland AG 2021
S. Cousty, S. Laurencin-Dalicieux (eds.), *Drug-Induced Oral Complications*,
https://doi.org/10.1007/978-3-030-66973-7_6

or decrease in OPG leads to increased bone resorption. Monoclonal antibody denosumab is a RANK-L inhibitor with antiresorptive and antiangiogenic properties. This drug can inhibit osteoclast function, decrease bone resorption, and increase bone density and is therefore used in the management of the following conditions:

- Osteoporosis (Prolia®).
- Prevention of skeletal-related events in adults with bone metastases from solid tumors (pathological fractures, bone radiation therapy, spinal cord compression, or bone surgery) (Xgeva®).
- Treatment of adults and skeletally mature adolescents with unresectable benign bone tumors (such as giant cell bone tumors) or when surgical resection is likely to result in severe morbidity (Xgeva®).
- Malignancy-associated hypercalcemia (Xgeva®).

Denosumab is administered as a subcutaneous injection once every 4 weeks (Xgeva®) or every 6 months to prevent osteoporosis-related fractures (Prolia®). Unlike bisphosphonates, there is no long-term accumulation of this molecule in the bone matrix; it is considered that normal bone remodeling is restored 3–6 months after treatment discontinuation.

2.2 Antiangiogenic Agents

Antiangiogenic agents inhibit the development of novel blood vessels by blocking the angiogenesis signaling cascade. They are used in the treatment of gastrointestinal tumors, renal cell carcinomas, neuroendocrine tumors, and others, and help prevent tumor invasion of vessels and metastases. There are mainly two types of drugs that can be used.

2.2.1 Bevacizumab
Tumor cells release several pro-angiogenic factors that stimulate endothelial cell proliferation and migration. One of these factors, the vascular endothelial growth factor (VEGF), is the target of monoclonal antibody bevacizumab.

2.2.2 Sunitinib and Sorafenib
The VEGF pathway can also be blocked by inhibiting its tyrosine kinase receptors. Sunitinib and sorafenib are small molecules that inhibit cellular signaling by targeting tyrosine kinase receptors, limiting tumor angiogenesis.

A few cases of ONJ induced by everolimus and sirolimus, two mammalian target of rapamycin (mTor) inhibitors used in oncology, have been reported since 2013, but further investigation is necessary in this field.

ICD	Brand name	Route	Primary indication
Bisphosphonates/1st generation			
Etidronate	Didronel®	Oral	Osteoporosis
Clodronate	Clastoban®	Oral/IV	Oncology
	Lytos®	Oral	Oncology
Tiludronate	Skelid®	Oral	Paget's disease
Bisphosphonates/2nd generation			
Pamidronate	Aredia®	IV	Oncology, Paget's disease
Alendronate	Fosamax®	Oral	Osteoporosis
	Fosavance®	Oral	Osteoporosis
Bisphosphonates/3rd generation			
Risedronate	Actonel®	Oral	Osteoporosis, Paget's disease
Ibandronate	Boniva®/Bonviva®	Oral/IV	Osteoporosis
	Bondronat®	IV	Oncology
Zolendronate	Zometa®	IV	Oncology
	Reclast®/Aclasta®	IV	Osteoporosis, Paget's disease
RANKL inhibitors			
Denosumab	Xgeva®	SQ	Oncology
	Prolia®	SQ	Osteoporosis

ICD	Brand name	Route	Primary indication
Tyrosine kinase inhibitors			
Sunitinib	Sutent®	Oral	Oncology
Sorafenib	Nexavar®	Oral	Oncology
Anti-VEGF			
Bevacizumab	Avastin®	IV	Oncology
mTor inhibitors			
Sirolimus	Rapamune®	Oral	Oncology
Everolimus	Afinitor®	Oral	Oncology

3 Pathophysiology of MRONJ

The pathophysiology of osteonecrosis of the jaw has not yet been completely elucidated. Several hypothesis have been put forward, in an attempt to explain its unique localization to the jaws, but most authors seem to agree that ONJ is a multifactorial condition. Among these hypotheses are: altered bone remodeling and resorption, inflammation or infection, angiogenesis inhibition, constant microtrauma, suppression of immunity, soft tissue BPs toxicity, vitamin D deficiency, terminal vascularization of the mandible, and specific oral flora.

3.1 Proposed Hypothesis

3.1.1 Inhibition of Osteoclastic Bone Resorption and Remodeling

Bisphosphonates and other antiresorptive drugs such as RANK-L inhibitors have a direct effect on osteoclasts, limiting their differentiation, function, and increasing apoptosis. This significantly attenuates bone remodeling and reduces skeletal-related complications in patients with osteoporosis or malignant diseases. Osteoclast differentiation and function is essential in all bony structures for bone healing and remodeling. It seems, however, that osteonecrosis occurs primarily within the alveolar bone of the maxilla and mandible. The increased remodeling rate observed in the jaws' alveolar bone could explain the increased predisposition for the development of ONJ in these sites. The fact that the incidence of ONJ is similar with BPs and RANK-L inhibitors such as denosumab enhances the essential role of bone remodeling inhibition. The main difference between these two molecules is that RANK-L inhibitors have a significantly shorter half-life than bisphosphonates, leading to a rapid reversibility of their antiresorptive effects.

3.1.2 Inflammation/Infection

Only a small number of patients treated with antiresorptives for malignant diseases develop an osteonecrosis of the jaws (0.8–12%), which means that other systemic and local risk factors must be taken into account. One of the best-known risk factors of ONJ is tooth extraction, which increases local inflammation and bone turnover. However, the indication leading to the extraction is often the existence of periapical or periodontal infection or inflammation. Several animal studies have demonstrated that the association of inflammation or bacterial infection with a systemic antiresorptive is sufficient for the development of osteonecrosis of the jaw. The role of infection and inflammation in the onset of ONJ justifies the implementation of dental screening and elimination of oral infections prior to treatment.

3.1.3 Inhibition of Angiogenesis

Inhibition of angiogenesis is a leading hypothesis of ONJ physiopathology since osteonecrosis derives from an interruption in blood supply, leading to an avascular necrosis. Antiangiogenic therapies play a major part in ONJ disease processes, but bisphosphonates, especially aminobisphosphonates also inhibit neovascularization. Denosumab has not been linked to an antiangiogenic effect, ruling out the possibility of angiogenesis inhibition as a sole cause of ONJ.

3.1.4 Other Hypotheses

Soft Tissue Toxicity

One of the first hypothesis in ONJ pathophysiology was the possibility of direct soft tissue toxicity of BPs. In vitro studies have shown that second- and third-generation BPs can increase apoptosis or decrease proliferation of multiple cell types. However, the fact that BP's extraosseous concentration is minimal (they are excreted renally after only a few hours in the blood stream) and the fact that no soft tissue toxicity has been reported with denosumab undermine this hypothesis.

Immune Dysfunction

Innate or acquired immunity dysfunction can promote ONJ development. Clinical studies have shown that patients with impaired immune function, such as patients treated with chemotherapy and steroids, seem to be more subject to ONJ.

3.2 Risk Factors

3.2.1 Medication-Related Risk Factors

MRONJ frequency depends mainly on three criteria: therapeutic indications (osteoporosis/osteopenia or malignancy), type of medication (BP and non-BP), and duration of the treatment. MRONJ risk among cancer patients is higher than for patients treated for osteoporosis or other benign conditions (approximately 70% of reported ONJ occur in cancer patients).

Among bisphosphonates, amino-BPs, especially third-generation BPs such as zolendronate, present the highest risk of inducing osteonecrosis (0.7–6.7%). This can be explained by the administration mode: IV treatment provides much higher doses of BPs compared to oral treatment. The risk for ONJ among cancer patients exposed to denosumab is comparable to the risk of ONJ in patients exposed to zolendronate.

The incidence of ONJ among patients treated with antiangiogenic drugs (tyrosine kinase inhibitors and monoclonal antibodies targeting VEGF) is difficult to estimate since actual data is mostly based on case reports. There seems however to exist a cumulative toxic effect when these drugs are associated to bisphosphonates, significantly increasing the risk of developing ONJ. The incidence of ONJ in patients treated with antiangiogenic agent bevacizumab is estimated around 0.2%, but can increase to 0.9% when associated with zoledronic acid.

The risk of developing ONJ among osteoporotic patients exposed to oral, IV BPs, or denosumab exists, but remains very low. Incidence of ONJ among patients treated with IV bisphosphonates or denosumab for osteoporosis is estimated at 0.017–0.04%, whereas for patients exposed to oral BPs it varies between 0.004% and 0.2%.

Regardless of indications for therapy, the duration of BP or antiresorptive therapy is considered a risk factor for developing ONJ. The cumulative dose, determined by the number of received injections and the potency of the administered molecule, must be taken into account. For patients receiving zolendronate or denosumab, the risk of developing ONJ doubles after 2–3 years of treatment. For patients receiving oral bisphosphonate therapy to manage osteoporosis, the incidence of ONJ seems to be also linked to treatment duration; it increases over time from near 0 at initiation of treatment to 0.21% after 4 or more years of BP exposure.

3.2.2 Local Factors

Oral Surgery

Dentoalveolar surgery is considered a major risk factor for developing MRONJ, since more than 50% of ONJ develop following tooth extraction. Estimates for developing osteonecrosis after dentoalveolar surgery among cancer patients exposed to intravenous BPs ranges from 1.6 to 14.8% and is around 0.5% among patients exposed to oral bisphosphonates. For patients exposed to antiresorptive drugs, the risk of developing ONJ after tooth extraction is still to be determined.

Anatomic Factors

The incidence of ONJ is higher in the mandible (73%) than in the maxilla (22.5%), but both jaws can be involved in 4.5% of cases. Special attention should be paid to removable prosthetic overdenture wearers under bisphosphonate therapy.

Concomitant Oral Disease

Dental inflammation and infection are well-known risk factors, present in 50% of reported ONJ in cancer patients. However, as the most common treatment for periapical or periodontal infection is tooth extraction, preexisting dental disease may confound the link between tooth extraction and incidence of osteonecrosis.

3.2.3   Systemic Factors

Age and sex have been reported as risk factors for MRONJ. Over 70% of patients with ONJ are female, with a mean age of 66.5 years. Corticosteroid treatment and antiangiogenic agents, when taken concomitantly with antiresorptive drugs, are associated with an increased risk of ONJ. For some authors, diabetes and tobacco also favor ONJ development.

3.2.4   Genetic Factors

Some reports seem to indicate the existence of a genetic predisposition to the occurrence of ONJ. Genetic analyses have shown that several single-nucleotide polymorphisms (SNPs) located within gene regions associated with bone turnover, collagen formation, or metabolic bone diseases are associated with medication-related osteonecrosis.

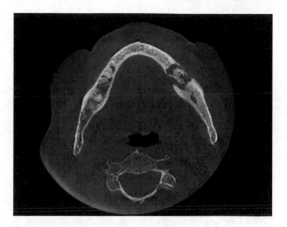

Fig. 1 Radiological examination of MRONJ: bone lysis and bony sequestra in an 81-year-old patient

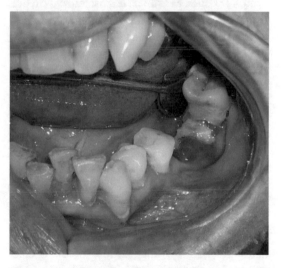

Fig. 2 Clinical examination of MRONJ: gingival ulceration and bone exposure in an 81-year-old patient

4   Clinical Presentation

In order to establish a diagnosis of MRONJ, the following characteristics must be present (Figs. 1 and 2):

- Ongoing or previous treatment with antiangiogenic or antiresorptive drugs.
- Exposed bone or bone that can be probed through an intraoral or extraoral fistula in the maxillofacial region, persisting for more than 8 weeks.
- No patient history of radiation therapy or manifest metastatic disease to the jaws.

It is important to highlight that exposed necrotic bone is not an absolute criterion for the diagnosis of ONJ, but solely one of the possible manifestations. According to Fedele et al., only 76% of the MRONJ are diagnosed; the 24% remaining ONJ are not diagnosed because of nonvisible necrotic bone in the oral cavity.

There are several staging systems for medication-related osteonecrosis of the jaws, mostly based on clinical presentation of the disease. Ruggiero et al. proposed in 2006 a clinical classification of ONJ with three different stages (1, 2, and 3), depending on the severity of the patient's symptoms. This classification was complemented by the American Association of Oral and Maxillofacial Surgeons (AAOMS) in 2009 since, in some cases, patients may develop symptoms of pain prior to the development of radiographic changes suggestive of osteonecrosis or clinical evidence of exposed bone.

4.1 Staging of MRONJ

At risk category: No apparent necrotic bone in patients who have been treated with antiresorptive drugs.

Stage 0: No clinical evidence of necrotic bone, associated with nonspecific clinical findings and symptoms such as pain or osteosclerosis. An oral fistula may be present at this stage.

Stage 1: Exposed bone that is asymptomatic, with no signs of swelling, inflammation, or infection in the adjacent or regional soft tissues.

Stage 2: Exposed bone with associated infection, resulting in pain, soft tissue inflammation and swelling, sometimes purulent drainage.

Stage 3: Exposed bone associated with pain, infection, soft tissue inflammation, swelling, and one or more of the following: pathologic fracture, extraoral cutaneous fistula, osteolysis extending to the sinus floor or the inferior mandibular border. The infection at this stage is difficult to manage with oral or intravenous antibiotic therapy, and because of the greater volume of necrotic bone, surgical therapy is often necessary.

Radiological examination completes the clinical examination helping with diagnosis and follow-up of MRONJ.

Orthopantomography is a simple examination associated with a low radiation dose, allowing the observation of persisting alveolar sockets, lamina dura sclerosis, bone lysis, or bony sequestra. 3D imaging techniques, such as cone beam computed tomography (CBCT) or computed tomography scan (CT scan), are also useful as they can help detect early changes in bone structure. At the first stage of ONJ, an increased bone density of the alveolar bone region can be observed, with a markedly thickened lamina dura. At stage 2,

osteosclerosis can extend to the basal bone and may be associated with the following signs: prominence of the inferior alveolar nerve canal, periosteal reaction, sinusitis, sequestra formation, and oroantral fistula. At stage 3, in addition to the previous radiological signs, a pathologic mandible fracture can be detected and osteolysis can also extend to the sinus floor.

Differential diagnoses for this condition include alveolar osteitis, periapical pathology, chronic sclerosing osteomyelitis, fibro-osseous lesions, and sarcoma, among others.

5 Treatment of MRONJ

The treatment of osteonecrosis of the jaws is generally difficult, especially since the optimal therapy strategy is still to be established. For this reason, the cornerstone of treatment lies in a preventive approach.

5.1 Prevention Strategies

Dental screening and appropriate dental treatment are essential to reduce the risk of ONJ in patients before initiating the administration of antiresorptive or antiangiogenic therapy and also during treatment. As such, treatment planning for patients who may be prescribed antiresorptive or antiangiogenic therapy should include consultation with a dental professional in order to perform a meticulous examination of the oral cavity and a radiographic assessment. It is important to identify both active and potential infections to prevent future invasive dental procedures and their complications. Periodontal disease, periapical pathology, presence of root fragments, caries, and partially embedded teeth represent potential infection sites. Denture stability should also be assessed since repeated soft tissue trauma may lead to bone exposure. Finally, patients should be informed of the risks of ONJ and educated as to the importance of oral hygiene, regular dental evaluations, and the necessity to report any pain, swelling, or exposed bone. The European

Medicines Agency (EMA) recently undertook a review of the effectiveness of risk minimization measures regarding the risk of osteonecrosis of the jaw with bisphosphonates and denosumab. This has resulted in a recommendation that reinforced safety messages be reflected in the product information (which contains the SmPC and package leaflet) for these products, as well as introduction of a patient reminder card, giving details of precautions aiming at minimizing the risk of ONJ.

The preventive strategy depends on the administration mode of the antiresorptive drug (oral or IV).

5.1.1 Patients About to Initiate Intravenous Antiresorptive or Antiangiogenic Treatment for Cancer Therapy

The treatment objective for this category of patients is to minimize the risk of developing osteonecrosis of the jaws. As dentoalveolar surgery is one of the main triggering factors for ONJ, initiation of the treatment should be delayed until dental health is optimized and the mucosa of the extraction sites has healed (2–3 weeks), provided the patient's general health allows it. This decision is made in conjunction with the dental practitioner, the oncologist, and the other specialists involved in the care of the patient.

Non-restorable teeth and those with poor prognosis should be extracted, as well as partially embedded teeth. Embedded teeth entirely covered by bone and soft tissue without communication with the oral cavity should be left undisturbed. Conservative endodontic and prosthodontic therapies of teeth with good prognosis should be completed. Periodontal disease should be treated and tooth mobility managed according to the patient's hygiene and compliance; stabilization splints can be used for teeth with Grades 1–2 mobility in patients with good dental hygiene, whereas extractions may be necessary in patients with poor dental hygiene. Mucosal trauma must be prevented in patients with full or partial dentures, especially along the lingual flange region.

5.1.2 Asymptomatic Patients Receiving Intravenous Antiresorptive or Antiangiogenic Treatment for Cancer Therapy

A periodic clinical follow-up every 4–6 months is necessary; its frequency depends on the medical administration, the number of risk factors, and oral health status. An orthopantomography should be performed every 6–12 months for radiographic evidence of ONJ, such as osteosclerosis, osteolysis, widened periodontal ligament spaces. The maintenance of a good oral hygiene is essential to prevent dental infections that may require dentoalveolar surgery. Conservative treatment and extractions limited to teeth with Grade 3 mobility or endodontic-periodontal lesions should be favored. If extraction cannot be avoided, it should be completed with the minimum bone injury and under antibiotic prophylaxis. The latter must be extended until mucosa of the surgical site has healed. Penicillin is the first choice, but a combination of quinolones–metronidazole or erythromycin–metronidazole can be used in the event of penicillin allergy. Placement of dental implants should be avoided.

5.1.3 Patients About to Initiate Antiresorptive Treatment for Osteoporosis

Preventive measures are similar to those regarding oncology patients. Patients should be instructed of the risk of developing ONJ and the importance of oral hygiene and health. The risk associated with oral bisphosphonate treatment is 10–100 times smaller compared to IV treatment in oncology, but increases if the duration of therapy exceeds four years. Other clinical risk factors must be taken into account, such as concomitant antiangiogenic or corticosteroid treatment.

Asymptomatic Patients Receiving Antiresorptive Treatment for Osteoporosis

- *Patients treated with oral aminobisphosphonates for less than 4 years without risk factors.*
- For patients receiving oral medication, all dental procedures can be undertaken and mod-

ification or delay of surgery are not necessary. Implant placement is possible provided the patient is given adequate information regarding the possible risk of implant failure and ONJ if the antiresorptive treatment is continued. A periodic clinical and radiological follow-up is necessary every 6–12 months.

- *Patients treated with oral aminobisphosphonates for less than 4 years with risk factors or for more than 4 years.*
- Invasive surgery should be avoided if possible and antibiotic prophylaxis for surgery procedures is advised. Implant placement is possible, but the patient should be informed about the possibility of short- and long-term loss of dental implants and ONJ risk.
- There is not enough data to support the cessation of medical treatment in patients with osteoporosis or malignancy before oral surgical procedures. If the patient's condition allows it, the prescribing provider could consider discontinuation of the oral bisphosphonate for at least 2 months prior to oral surgery; osseous healing should be obtained before restarting the bisphosphonate.

5.2 Treatment of Medication-Related Osteonecrosis of the Jaw

Treatment of ONJs is a challenge since an effective and appropriate MRONJ therapy is still to be determined. As with preventive strategies, a multidisciplinary team approach, including a dentist, an oncologist, and an oral/maxillofacial surgeon, is necessary to evaluate and decide the best treatment strategy for the patient. According to the American Association of Oral and Maxillofacial Surgeons (AAOMS), treatment goals are preservation of quality of life through pain and infection control, as well as prevention of bone necrosis extension and prioritization and support of continued oncologic treatment in patients receiving IV antiresorptive and antiangiogenic therapy. Therefore, the choice between a conservative or surgical approach is not always easy and is specific to each case.

We present here the stage-specific treatment strategies recommended by the AAOMS:

5.2.1 Stage 0
Treatment should be symptomatic, based on antiseptic, analgesic, antibiotic, and antiphlogistic medication. Local risk factors such as caries and periodontal disease must be managed. Close follow-up is required since the disease can progress to a higher stage.

5.2.2 Stage 1
In the presence of exposed necrotic bone or fistula, an antiseptic rinse (chlorhexidine 0.12%) should be prescribed. In the absence of healing after 8 weeks, a surgical debridement approach can be considered.

5.2.3 Stage 2
A combination of oral antimicrobial rinses and antibiotics is prescribed since the colonization of exposed bone by oral pathogens is frequent. Usually, these are sensitive to the penicillin group of antibiotics, but microbial cultures should be analyzed to better adapt the antibiotic therapy. Surgical debridement can be performed to reduce the volume of colonized, necrotic bone and stimulate soft tissue healing.

5.2.4 Stage 3
Surgical debridement is necessary, in combination with antibiotic therapy. Large resections or segmental osteotomies are recommended for severe cases and may require perioperative reconstruction. If invasive surgery cannot improve the patient's quality of life, a conservative approach is adopted, in order to control symptoms and to prevent the osteonecrosis progression.

The most recent systematic review by Ramada et al. demonstrates that a conservative approach ensures good results at early stages, but disparate results at more advanced stages. Surgical approach presents more inconstant results at all stages. Furthermore, statistical analysis showed a significantly higher prevalence of completely healed sites in patients who followed a "drug-holiday" protocol.

Bibliography

Aghaloo T, Hazboun R, Tetradis S. Pathophysiology of osteonecrosis of the jaws. Oral Maxillofac Surg Clin North Am. 2015;27(4):489–96.

Bedogni A, Fusco V, Agrillo A, Campisi G. Learning from experience. Proposal of a refined definition and staging system for bisphosphonate-related osteonecrosis of the jaw (BRONJ). Oral Dis. 2012;18(6):621–3.

deBoissieu P, Gaboriau L, Morel A, Trenque T. Bisphosphonate-related osteonecrosis of the jaw: data from the French national pharmacovigilance database. Fundam Clin Pharmacol. 2016;30(5):450–8.

Dodson TB. The frequency of medication-related osteonecrosis of the jaw and its associated risk factors. Oral Maxillofac Surg Clin North Am. 2015;27(4):509–16.

Fantasia JE. The role of antiangiogenic therapy in the development of osteonecrosis of the jaw. Oral Maxillofac Surg Clin North Am. 2015;27(4):547–53.

Fedele S, Bedogni G, Scoletta M, Favia G, Colella G, Agrillo A, et al. Up to a quarter of patients with osteonecrosis of the jaw associated with antiresorptive agents remain undiagnosed. Br J Oral Maxillofac Surg. 2015;53(1):13–7.

Japanese Allied Committee on Osteonecrosis of the Jaw, Yoneda T, Hagino H, Sugimoto T, Ohta H, Takahashi S, et al. Antiresorptive agent-related osteonecrosis of the jaw: position paper 2017 of the Japanese Allied Committee on Osteonecrosis of the Jaw. J Bone Miner Metab. 2017;35(1):6–19.

Khan AA, Morrison A, Hanley DA, Felsenberg D, McCauley LK, O'Ryan F, et al. Diagnosis and management of osteonecrosis of the jaw: a systematic review and international consensus. J Bone Miner Res. 2015;30(1):3–23.

Marx RE. Pamidronate (Aredia) and zoledronate (Zometa) induced avascular necrosis of the jaws: a growing epidemic. J Oral Maxillofac Surg. 2003;61(9):1115–7.

Parretta E, Sottosanti L, Sportiello L, Rafaniello C, Potenza S, D'Amato S, et al. Bisphosphonate-related osteonecrosis of the jaw: an Italian post-marketing surveillance analysis. Expert Opin Drug Saf. 2014;13(Suppl 1):S31–40.

Ramaglia L, Guida A, Iorio-Siciliano V, Cuozzo A, Blasi A, Sculean A. Stage-specific therapeutic strategies of medication-related osteonecrosis of the jaws: a systematic review and meta-analysis of the drug suspension protocol. Clin Oral Investig. 2018;22(2):597–615.

Rosella D, Papi P, Giardino R, Cicalini E, Piccoli L, Pompa G. Medication-related osteonecrosis of the jaw: clinical and practical guidelines. J Int Soc Prev Community Dent. 2016;6(2):97–104.

Ruggiero S, Gralow J, Marx RE, Hoff AO, Schubert MM, Huryn JM, et al. Practical guidelines for the prevention, diagnosis, and treatment of osteonecrosis of the jaw in patients with cancer. J Oncol Pract. 2006;2(1):7–14.

Ruggiero SL, Dodson TB, Assael LA, Landesberg R, Marx RE, Mehrotra B, et al. American Association of Oral and Maxillofacial Surgeons position paper on bisphosphonate-related osteonecrosis of the jaws—2009 update. J Oral Maxillofac Surg. 2009;67(5 Suppl):2–12.

Ruggiero SL, Dodson TB, Fantasia J, Goodday R, Aghaloo T, Mehrotra B, et al. American Association of Oral and Maxillofacial Surgeons position paper on medication-related osteonecrosis of the jaw—2014 update. J Oral Maxillofac Surg. 2014;72(10):1938–56.

Drug-Induced Oral Bleeding

Cedric Mauprivez and Sébastien Laurence

Drug-induced oral bleedings are numerous and may be categorized according to the manner they impact hemostasis. This chapter will focus on oral bleeding that is caused primarily by antithrombotic drugs.

Postoperative bleeding complications after oral surgery occurred significantly more often in patients under antithrombotic therapy than in the control cases without antiplatelet and anticoagulation medication. Antithrombotic therapy has evolved considerably in recent years with the arrival of new drugs. Two novel antiplatelet agents, prasugrel and ticagrelor, have been used since 2010. Three novel oral anticoagulant drugs with selective and specific action on the activated factors II and X, known as direct oral anticoagulants, were released: dabigatran in 2008, rivaroxaban in 2009, and apixaban in 2012.

For each of these drugs, therapeutic progress is advanced: greater efficacy for new antiplatelet agents with a reduced number of nonresponders, a broad therapeutic range, and the unnecessity of biological monitoring for new oral anticoagulants. In addition, patients with high risk of thrombotic events, especially in the elderly, receive a combined antithrombotic therapy (combination of two antiplatelet agents or a combination of an antiplatelet agent and an oral anticoagulant).

The continuation of antithrombotic therapy prior to surgery ensures the prevention of the risk of thrombosis. In return, this approach increases the risk of perioperative bleeding.

1 Antiplatelet Agents

Antiplatelet agents (APAs) are indicated for secondary prevention in atheromatous disease to prevent the occurrence of cardiovascular events. Antiplatelet monotherapy (aspirin or clopidogrel) is recommended in patients with acute coronary syndromes, ischemic cerebrovascular accidents, or peripheral obstructive artery disease. Dual antiplatelet therapy (aspirin and clopidogrel or prasugrel or ticagrelor) is justified in cases of major risk of thrombosis, especially after myocardial infarction. Aspirin alone is recommended for primary prevention when cardiovascular risk is particularly high in patients with diabetes.

GP IIb/IIIa antagonists (abciximab, eptifibatide, tirofiban) indicated in the initial management of acute coronary syndromes are prescribed in hospital during emergency care.

Conventional APAs include:

Acetylsalicylic acid or aspirin blocks irreversibly the cyclooxygenase-1 (COX-1) of the platelet and inhibits the production of thromboxane A2 (TXA2) (a potent vasoconstrictor and inducer of platelet aggregation). The inhibition of COX-1

C. Mauprivez (✉) · S. Laurence
Oral Surgery, Dental Faculty, Reims, France
e-mail: cedric.mauprivez@univ-reims.fr

© Springer Nature Switzerland AG 2021
S. Cousty, S. Laurencin-Dalicieux (eds.), *Drug-Induced Oral Complications*,
https://doi.org/10.1007/978-3-030-66973-7_7

is complete under low-dose aspirin (75–160 mg/day) or after a loading dose of 325 mg. Daily doses above 100 mg in clinical practice do not increase the antiplatelet effect but increase the risk of spontaneous gastrointestinal bleeding. After discontinuation of aspirin, platelet aggregation normalizes within 5–7 days (on average 10% of platelets per day). Aspirin is the most widely used antiplatelet agent. It is marketed either alone or in combination with dipyridamole antiplatelet agents (APAs), clopidogrel or pravastatin.

All patients do not respond to aspirin with the same intensity. The rate of low responders to aspirin is around 6% of the population and is particularly significant in patients with type 1 diabetes and in females.

Dipyridamole slows down the reuptake of adenosine monophosphate (AMP) by platelets. It is also described as cyclic AMP (cAMP) inhibitor. Dipyridamole is marketed alone at a dose of 75 mg, 150 mg, or 200 mg combined with 25 mg of aspirin. The clinical efficacy of monotherapy dipyridamole is low.

Thienopyridines, including ticlopidine, clopidogrel, and prasugrel, inhibit irreversibly the P2Y12 purinergic ADP receptor, a factor for activation and platelet. Clopidogrel is currently the most prescribed thienopyridine, because it is more potent than ticlopidine with better pharmacokinetics (one dose daily instead of twice *per* day) and a better safety profile (rare cases of leukopenia and thrombocytopenia). Clopidogrel is a prodrug that requires first a hepatic biotransformation at the level of CYP 450. Clopidogrel has been used since 1998, at a dose of 75 mg daily. In monotherapy, clopidogrel has demonstrated superiority over aspirin only in the secondary prevention of transient ischemic attacks and ischemic cerebral vascular accident. The modes of action of aspirin and clopidogrel are different, and their combination suggests a high antithrombotic efficacy. The superiority of the dual therapy compared with aspirin alone was demonstrated in two situations: patients with myocardial infarction less than 1 year ago and after coronary revascularization. Several randomized studies have shown the benefits of dual therapy during the first 6–12 months after the placement of drug-eluting stents or a venous bypass, with a significant reduction in the rates of stent thrombosis, better maintenance of the permeability of vein graft, as well as reduced mortality. The optimal duration of dual therapy remains controversial. The antiplatelet activity of clopidogrel is subject to a large individual variability with a rate of nonresponders estimated at 12–35%. Several phenomena are involved: a genetic polymorphism, drug interactions (such as atorvastatin and omeprazole), type 1 diabetes, kidney failure, and old age.

Since 2010, two novels APAs are marketed:

Prasugrel is a third-generation thienopyridine, which has two essential advantages compared to ticlopidine and clopidogrel: early onset of action (30 min post-dose) and a higher potent activity. Prasugrel blocks the P2Y12 receptor sensitive to ADP, irreversibly, like ticlopidine and clopidogrel, but with a less variable and more predictive platelet inhibition. Prasugrel is used with a 60 mg loading dose and a maintenance dose of 10 mg 1 time/day. Prasugrel is more effective than clopidogrel) in terms of protection against myocardial infarction and stent thrombosis, but it exhibits more bleeding episodes. Prasugrel is particularly effective in diabetic patients and in nonresponders to clopidogrel. The rate of nonresponders to prasugrel is only 3%. Prasugrel is indicated in combination with acetylsalicylic acid for the prevention of atherothrombotic events in patients with acute coronary syndrome treated with primary or delayed percutaneous coronary intervention.

Ticagrelor, marketed since 2010, is an antiplatelet agent of a new chemical class, the family of cyclo-pentyl-triazolo-pyrimidines. It is a direct and reversible platelet P2Y12 receptor inhibitor. This is not a prodrug and it does not need to be metabolized to be active. Pharmacodynamic studies have shown that ticagrelor has a more powerful, faster platelet inhibition potency and with less individual variability compared to clopidogrel. Ticagrelor is used at a dose of 90 mg, 2 times/day after a loading dose of 180 mg.

Ticagrelor, in combination with aspirin, is indicated for the prevention of atherothrombotic events in adult patients with acute coronary syndrome, including medically treated patients and those treated with percutaneous coronary intervention or coronary artery bypass surgery.

1.1 Risks of Oral Bleeding with Antiplatelet Agents

The average risks of bleeding after dentoalveolar surgery in patients without interruption of antiplatelet therapy monotherapy (aspirin or clopidogrel) and bitherapy (aspirin and clopidogrel) are estimated at 2.56% (in case of monotherapy) and 16.37% (in case of biotherapy) (Table 1). In all clinical studies, there is no severe bleeding complications. In case of dual therapy, the incidence of bleeding with the aspirin + dipyridamole combination is similar to that observed with aspirin alone. However, in case of the aspirin + clopidogrel combination, the risk of bleeding during the immediate postoperative period is higher in the case of dual therapy compared to aspirin alone (RR 28, $p < 0.001$) and clopidogrel (RR 24, $p < 0.001$).

No severe or delayed bleeding is reported. A simple surgical hemostasis combining local hemostatic and sutures can be used to effectively control the risk of perioperative bleeding.

Furthermore, studies have shown the occurrence of thrombotic events within a period of 1–3 months, following the discontinuation of the dual therapy (discontinuation of clopidogrel and continuation of aspirin) in stent patients. This raises the question of a possible "prothrombotic rebound" upon discontinuation of clopidogrel, a deleterious effect also mentioned with aspirin, but whose physiopathology is still unclear.

All clinical studies show that dental extractions and dental implant placement can be performed with aspirin or clopidogrel monotherapy and in combination, without stopping APAs. No data has been published with prasugrel or ticagrelor. No laboratory test are currently available to evaluate or predict the risk of surgical bleeding in

Table 1 Management of dentoalveolar procedure (dental extraction, dental implant) in patient undergoing antiplatelet agents

Study	Without stopping antiplatelets agents					Control (no antithrombotic drugs)	
	Bitherapy (aspirin AND clopidogrel)		Monotherapy (aspirin OR clopidogrel)				
	Bleeding event(s) (n,%)	Total patients (N)	Bleeding event(s) (n,%)	Total patients (N)		Bleeding event(s) (n,%)	Total patients (N)
Ardekian 2000	–	–	2	19		4	20
Madan 2005	–	–	1	51		–	–
Garnier 2007	–	–	1	52		–	
Krishnan 2008	–	–	0	32		0	50
Canigral 2010	4	10	1	27		–	–
Napenas 2009	0	28	0	14		–	–
Lillis 2011							
– bleeding<24 h	22	–	2	–		2	*532*
– bleeding≥24 h	0	33	0	78		0	532
Park 2012	2	100	–	–		0	100
TOTAL	*28 (16.37)*[a]	*171*	*7 (2.56)*[a]	*273*		*6 (0.85)*[a]	*702*

[a]minor bleeding, no severe bleedings were reported
bolditalic values represent the average risk of bleeding: number of event and percentage

Without interruption or modifying antiplatelet therapy:			
	OR	[95% confidence interval]	*P* values
Monotherapy vs. no antithrombotic drugs	3.00	[1.00–9.01]	≤0.05
Bitherapy vs. no antithrombotic drugs	19.16	[7.81–47.01]	≤0.001
Bitherapy vs. monotherapy	6.39	[2.73–14.95]	≤0.001

patients on an antiplatelet agent. Conventional hemostatic measures (sutures + mechanical compression of 30 min) are effective and sufficient to control postoperative bleeding in patients on aspirin or on clopidogrel with an acceptable residual postoperative bleeding rate of about 2–3%. For aspirin + clopidogrel dual therapy, local hemostasis combining sutures + compression seems to be not sufficient and the use of local hemostatis (collagen sponge, oxycellulose gauze, fibrin glue) is necessary.

The management of a bleeding complication is always based on a surgical revision of local hemostasis. No severe bleeding complications not controllable by local hemostasis measures is reported in the literature.

2   Antivitamins K

VKAs are indicated in the prevention of thromboembolic events from cardiac origin (atrial fibrillation, valvular heart disease, prosthetic valve disease, and acute coronary syndrome) and from venous (superficial and deep vein thrombosis, pulmonary embolism). VKAs are usually prescribed as a relay to initial heparin therapy, injectable anticoagulants, and more adjusted during the acute phase. Anticoagulants exert no direct action on a thrombus already formed or on ischemic tissue lesions. However, in cases where the thrombus is formed, the administration of anticoagulants aims to prevent the clot from growing and to prevent secondary thromboembolic complications, which could lead to serious after effects and could even be fatal. More than two-thirds of VKA prescriptions fall under cardiology (valvular disease, arrhythmias, and coronary syndromes), while less than 20% fall under venous thromboembolic disease. In the cardiological indications, treatment is most often prescribed for life. In the indications for VTE, treatment is usually shorter, schematically from 3 months to 1 year.

VKAs are characterized by a narrow therapeutic window, and therapeutic balance is sometimes difficult to obtain. For each patient, the required dosage of VKAs is variable and must be adjusted according to the results of the INR. Drug interactions, dietary habits, and concurrent illnesses must be clearly identified and monitored over time in order to adjust the VKA treatment. VKAs involve an increased risk of major bleeding. This is estimated at 3% per year. Such bleeding is first among iatrogenic accidents, with 13% of hospitalizations for adverse drug reactions. They are directly responsible for 0.6% of deaths per year recorded in patients on long-term treatment with VKA.

2.1   Pharmacology of VKAs

The anticoagulant action of VKA is an indirect action; it is linked to reduced hepatic synthesis of vitamin K-dependent coagulation factors (factors II, VII, IX, and X).

INR is used to monitor the effectiveness of VKAs. The target INR values are usually between 2 and 3 when the risk of thrombosis is moderate, between 3 and 4.5 when it is major. An INR value greater than 6 is associated with a significantly increased risk of spontaneous major bleeding. Patients with a high target INR (at most between 3.5 and 4.5) have a higher risk of spontaneous bleeding (minor, major) than those with a target INR between 2 and 3. There are three currently available VKAs.

Warfarin is the most frequently prescribed VKA worldwide. It is prescribed at a dose of 2 mg and 5 mg, at 1 dose per day. It is a coumarin derivative with a long half-life (35–45 h). The anticoagulant effect is maximal between 72 and 96 h following administration. The duration of action of a single dose of warfarin varies among individuals between 2 and 5 days (96–120 h).

Acenocoumarol is a fast acting and short duration VKA (24 h). This drug is administered 1–2 times daily. In case of a single dose, it is preferable for the dose to be taken in the evening in order to adjust the dosage as soon as possible after the INR results. However, the use of this VKA is not often prescribed because it has a higher risk of therapeutic instability.

Fluindione is the only indane-dione derivative. It is a long half-life compound (30 h) with an onset and a prolonged duration of action (48–72 h).

2.2 Risks of Oral Bleeding with VKAs

Nearly 10% of patients on VKA undergo surgery every year. Three clinical approaches are possible: to maintain the treatment, discontinue it, or relay it with heparin. The choice of the modality of management of VKAs in case of oral surgery depends primarily on the type of surgery envisaged (dentoalveolar or surgery with a high risk of bleeding). The second criterion is the presence or absence of local or general factors that might increase the risk of bleeding. The existence of several risk factors can lead to a situation with high bleeding risk (Tables 2 and 3).

For the patients undergoing dentoalveolar surgery, the risk of bleeding is low and easily controllable by a local hemostasis. Dental extractions and dental implants can be performed without interrupting VKAs (after checking the INR and verifying a value <4). The bleeding rate after dental extraction or dental implant placement in patients undergoing VKAs without discontinuation treatment is less than 10% according the literature (Table 2). In case of overdose (INR greater than 4), the surgical procedure has to be postponed. Corrective measures must be initiated immediately by the prescribing physician to bring the INR within the therapeutic range (skipping a dose, intake of Vitamin K, emergency hospitalization). Within the therapeutic range, the majority of observational studies indicate no positive correlation between preoperative INR value and the rate of incidence of post-extraction bleeding.

For surgical procedures with high risk of bleeding (i.e., sinus-lift, bone grafting), the discontinuation of VKA with or without relay heparin, depending on the risk of thrombosis for the patient, is recommended. The decision to temporarily discontinue VKA therapy must always be taken after consultation with the physician who prescribed the VKA.

For patients at low risk of thrombosis, discontinuing VKAs without replacement therapy can be proposed. For patients at a high risk of thrombosis, pre- and postoperative relay heparin is recommended.

Use of local hemostatics (tranexamic acid, gelatin sponge, collagen, oxycellulose gauze) in case of dental extraction(s) in patients) under VKAs must be systematic.

Many drugs interfere with VKAs. Some contribute to the occurrence of biological overdose (INR ≥ 4.0).

Co-prescription is a risk factor for imbalance in the intestinal flora and disruption of the endogenous synthesis of vitamin K, with a consequence of an imbalance of VKA therapy and an increased risk of bleeding. However, oral infection must be treated with the appropriate conventional antibiotics with close monitoring of the INR. It should be noted that antibiotic prophylaxis does not change the value of the INR. Miconazole is strictly contraindicated, including topical use. No azole antifungals are recommended. In patients treated with VKA, amphotericin B is the recommended antifungal for the treatment of oropharyngeal candidiasis.

For mild to moderate pain, the prescription of aspirin (at analgesic doses) is strictly contraindicated and that of NSAIDs is not recommended because bleeding risk could be severe and/or unpredictable severe systemic bleeding (gastrointestinal and intracranial bleeding). The administration of paracetamol is possible, but in the elderly, dosage adjustment (<2 g/day) and the prescription of an INR during the postoperative period are measures used to limit and detect the occurrence of any overdose. For moderate to severe pain, opiate derivatives (codeine, tramadol) may be prescribed.

The management of postoperative bleeding complications is mainly based on surgical revision and on the investigation of a local cause of the bleeding. Usefulness of biological glue is clinically relevant.

3 Direct Oral Anticoagulants

Since 2009, a new class of oral anticoagulants is available. These are selective direct oral anticoagulants (DOACs), either thrombin (anti-IIa) or activated factor X (anti-Xa) (Thean and Alberghini 2016). Their indications, limited at

Table 2 Management of dentoalveolar procedure (dental extraction, dental implant) in patients undergoing antivitamins K therapy

Study	No discontinuation of VKAs Preoperative INR < 4		Stopping of VKAs Preoperative INR < 2		Reducing dose of VKAs		Bridging therapy using LMWH		Control (no antithrombotic drugs)	
	Bleeding event(s) (n,%)	Total patients (N)	Bleeding event(s)	Total patients	Bleeding event(s)	Total patients	Bleeding event(s)	Total patients	Bleeding event(s) (n,%)	Total patients (N)
Al-Belasy 2003	5 (16.67)	30	–	–	–	–	–	–	0 (0.00)	10
Bacci 2010	7 (1.56)	449	–	–	–	–	–	–	4 (0.89)	449
Bacci 2011	2 (3.85)	52							3 (2.75)	109
Bajkin 2009	8 (7.34)	109	–	–	–	–	5	105	–	–
Bajkin 2015	7 (5.60)	125							1 (1.18)	85
Blinder 1999	13 (8.67)	150	–	–	–	–	–	–	–	–
Blinder 2001	30 (12.05)	249	–	–	–	–	–	–	–	–
Bodner 1998	2 (2.90)	69							–	–
Borea 1993	1 (6.67)	15	–	–	2	15	–	–	–	–
Broekema 2014	3 (9.38)	32	–	35	–	–	–	–	2 (1.94)	103
Cannon 2003	2 (5.71)	35	3	35	–	–	–	–	–	–
Carter 2003	3 (6.12)	49	–	–	–	–	–	–	–	–
Devani 1998	1 (3.03)	33	–	–	1	32	–	–	–	–
Eichhorn 2012	47 (7.38)	637							2 (0.70)	285
Evans 2002	15 (26.32)	57	7	52	–	–	–	–	–	–
Febbo 2016	9 (2.05)	439	–	–	2	32	–	–	0 (0.00)	439
Gaspar 1997	1 (6.67)	15	–	–	–	–	–	–	–	–
Halfpenny 2001	3 (7.50)	40	–	–	–	–	–	–	–	–
Karsl2011	6 (46.15)	13							3 (23.08)	13
Sacco 2007	6 (9.23)	65			10	66			–	–
Salam 2007	10 (6.67)	150	–	–	–	–	–	–	–	–
Zanon 2003	4 (1.60)	250			–	–			3 (1.20)	250
TOTAL	*185 (6.04)*	*3063*	*10 (8.70)*	*87*	*13 (11.50)*	*113*	*5 (4.76)*	*105*	*18 (1.03)*	*1743*

Without interruption or modifying antivitamins K therapy and with use of local hemostatic measures

	OR global	[95% confidence interval]	
			P values
VKAs vs. no antithrombotic drugs	1.71	[0.68–4.32]	≤ 0.30

bolditalic values represent the average risk of bleeding; number of event and percentage first to the prevention of the risk of venous thromboembolism after orthopedic surgery (total hip and knee replacement), were extended starting in 2012 to the prevention of thromboembolic events in patients with nonvalvular atrial fibrillation associated with one or more risk factors. DOACs have significant advantages over VKAs (current standard of care): the absence of food interaction, a limited number of drug interactions reflect a "more predictable" anticoagulant activity that makes it possible to administer them at a fixed dose (for each patient), and not to resort to biological monitoring. DOACs are contraindicated in patients with mitral stenosis or patients with prosthetic heart valves. DOACs are mainly used as an alternative to VKAs and/or LMWHs and are intended for a large population. The use of DOACs, since 2012, date of the beginning of their marketing, has increased year on year and has become important worldwide. Then, they have received increasing attention in the dental community.

3.1 Pharmacology of DAOCs

Four novel oral anticoagulants or direct oral anticoagulants (DOACs) have currently available for use worldwide. These are dabigatran, a direct thrombin inhibitor, and rivaroxaban, apixaban, and endoxaban, which are factor Xa inhibitors. They differ in dosing regimen (once or twice daily) and degree of renal elimination. In contrast to VKAs, DOACs have a short onset of action (peak plasma levels after 1–4 h) and a short half-life (5–17 h). Three DOACs compounds are currently marketed worldwide.

Dabigatran etexilate is a direct thrombin inhibitor (direct anti-IIa) whose inhibition is concentration dependent, competitive, highly selective, and reversible. This drug is available in three dosages: 75 mg, 110 mg, and 150 mg.

Rivaroxaban is a direct, competitive, and highly selective factor Xa inhibitor (direct anti-Xa). Its selectivity for factor Xa is more than 10,000 times that of other serine proteases (factors Va, IXa, XIa, thrombin, and activated protein C). The inhibition of factor Xa interrupts the intrinsic and extrinsic pathways of the blood coagulation cascade, thereby inhibiting the generation of thrombin and development of thrombi. Rivaroxaban does not inhibit thrombin (factor IIa) and it has no demonstrated effect on platelets. Rivaroxaban is available in three dosages: 10 mg, 15 mg, and 20 mg.

Apixaban, like rivaroxaban, is a direct selective inhibitor of factor Xa, with no activity on thrombin. No food interactions have been reported in the literature. Its renal elimination is low (25% in the active form). Apixaban is available in two dosages: 2.5 and 5 mg.

Currently, there is only one agent (idarucizumab) as a specific antidote targeted to reverse dabigatran.

3.2 Risks of Oral Bleeding with DOACs

Some clinical studies have evaluated the incidence of bleeding in dental patients taking DOACs alone and/or combined with antiplatelet therapy. The risk of bleeding after dental surgery is approximately of 10%.

In patients treated with DOACs, prescribing aspirin at high doses (1 g per dose or 3 g/day), NSAIDs (all), clarithromycin, or azole antifungals may increase the risk of bleeding.

Several perioperative approaches have been recommended, such as continuing DAOC, delaying invasive treatment as late as possible after the last DAOC dose, or discontinuing DAOCs for 24–48 h.

Based on the manufacturers' recommendations, one might consider it wise to ask the patient to omit a dose of a DOAC before the dentoalveolar procedure, in order to reduce the risk of bleeding. However, these guidelines for dental management of DOACs patients (written by nondental surgeon) proposed to discontinue anticoagulation therapy, because these authors overrate the potential risk of bleeding compared to thromboembolic complications.

The current guidelines of the European Heart Rhythm Association advise, when the intervention does carry "no clinically important bleeding

Table 3 Management of dental extraction in patients undergoing bitherapy (antivitamins K + antiplatelet agents)

Study	VKAs		Antiplatelet		VKAs + APP	
	Bleeding event(s)	Total patients	Bleeding event(s)	Total patients	Bleeding event(s)	Total patients
	(n,%)	(N)	(n,%)	(N)	(n,%)	(N)
Bajkin 2012	2	71	0	71	3	71
Morimoto 2008	7	134	2	87	2	49
Morimoto 2011	9	188	2	128	6	66
TOTAL	18 (4.58)[a]	393	4 (1.39)[a]	286	12 (6.45)[a]	186

[a]minor bleeding, no severe bleedings were reported
bolditalic values represent the average risk of bleeding: number of event and percentage

risk" and/or when adequate local hemostasis is possible, likesome dental procedures, to perform the procedure at trough level of the DOACs (i.e., 12 or 24 h after the last intake, depending on bid or qd dosing). Dental extraction at peak levels should be avoided.

According to the French Society of Oral Surgery, all dental extraction or dental implant placement should be performed without antithrombotic agent discontinuation. This approach is in accordance with the low incidence and severity of post-extraction/postimplantation bleeding reported in clinical studies (Table 4).

The data of these studies suggest that modifications of DAOC therapy for dental surgical procedures are unnecessary, but the use of local measures for hemostasis must be systematically required. Furthermore, the risk of bleeding in dental patients using DOACS is low with no major complications. However, the optimal periprocedural management of DOACs in oral surgery remains unclear. A preoperative INR in patients treated by DAOCs is useless. Currently, no biological test available in routine can predict a high risk of bleeding.

Local hemostasis (gelatin sponge, collagen, fibrin, or oxycellulose gauze) in addition to conventional measures (sutures and compression) are recommended to reduce the risk of post-extraction bleeding. Tranexamic acid and conventional measures are indicated in case of dental implant surgery (Figs. 1, 2, and 3).

4 Injectable Anticoagulants

The prevention and treatment of venous thromboembolism in surgery, medicine, and oncology is based on injectable anticoagulants. Duration of the thromboprophylaxis depends on the type of surgery and the patient's medical status.

4.1 Pharmacology of Injectable Anticoagulants

Injectable anticoagulants include standard or unfractionated heparin (UFH) and low-molecular-weight heparins (LMWH).

Heparin was discovered in 1916. It potentiates antithrombin (AT), a physiological inhibitor of factors Xa and IIa. There are two UFHs: heparin sodium for IV bolus injection or continuous administration by syringe pump and heparin calcium for SC injection at two doses given every 12 h or at three doses every 8 h. After IV injection, the elimination half-life of heparin is 90 min. The administration of UFH usually requires hospitalization and a strict protocol. The major side effect, besides the risk of bleeding, is the risk of heparin-induced thrombocytopenia (HIT). HIT is a thrombotic, immuno-allergic, rare but serious complication, involving the vital and functional prognosis, requiring immediate discontinuation of heparin. Its risk for patients on UFH is estimated at between 1% and 5%.

Table 4 Management of dentoalveolar procedure (dental extraction, dental implant) in patients undergoing direct oral anticoagulants

Study	No discontinuation of DOACs		Skipping last dose of DOACs		Multiple periprocedural schedule		Control		No antithrombotic drugs	
							Without interruption or modifying VKAs			
	Bleeding event(s) (n,%)	Total patients (N)	Bleeding event(s) (n,%)	Total patients (N)	Bleeding event(s) (n,%)	Total patients (N)	Bleeding event(s) (n,%)	Total patients (N)	Bleeding event(s) (n,%)	Total patients (N)
Clemm 2016	0 (0.00)	16	–	–	–	–	2 (6.66%)	30	3 (0.67)	447
Gómez-Moreno 2016a	2 (6.89)	29	–	–	–	–	–	–	2 (4.76)	42
Gómez-Moreno 2016b	1 (5.55)	18	–	–	–	–			2 (5.19)	39
Hanken 2015	6 (11.50)	52							2 (0.70)	285
Mauprivez 2016	7 (22.58)	31	–	–	–	–	5 (25.00)	20	–	–
Miclotte 2003	–	–	12 (46.15)	26	–	–	–	–	5 (19.23)	26
Patel 2017	–	–			15 (13.51)	111	–	–	–	–
Yagyuu 2017	4 (9.75)	41	–	–	–	–	5 (10.00%)	50	6 (11.11)	54
Zeevi 2017	7 (6.31)	111	–	–	–	–	–	–	–	–
TOTAL	*27 (9.06)*[a]	298					*12 (12.00)*[a]	100	*20 (2.24)*[a]	893

[a] minor bleeding, no severe bleedings were reported
bolditalic values represent the average risk of bleeding: number of event and percentage

Without interruption or modifying anticoagulant therapy:

	OR	[95% confidence interval]	P values
DOACs vs. no antithrombotic drugs	4.49	[2.44–8.27]	≤ 0.001
DOACs vs. VKAs	0.76	[0.37–1.56]	≤ 0.50

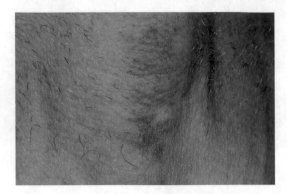

Fig. 1 Cutaneous hematoma of the neck, following oral surgery

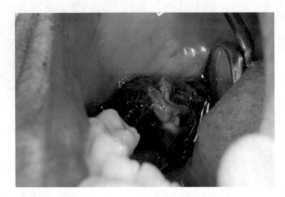

Fig. 2 Post-extraction blood clot, following surgery of the third molar

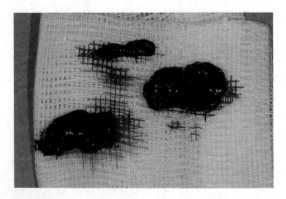

Fig. 3 Removal of voluminous blood clot

LMWHs are obtained by chemical depolymerization or enzymatic digestion of UFH chains. Decreasing the molecular weight of heparin chains (3–30,000 Da for UFHs and less than 8000 Da for LMWHs) gives LMWHs, compared with UFH, an anti-Xa activity that is predominant over anti-IIa activity (ratio ranging from 2 to 4 depending on the compounds) and a longer elimination half-life that makes it possible to reduce the number of daily injections to 1 or 2 injections per day. LMWHs have been marketed since 1985. There are main LMWH available: dalteparin sodium, enoxaparin sodium, tinzaparin sodium, and nadroparin calcium LMWHs. These have the same indications as UFHs and tend to replace them (better tolerance, reduced number of injections). However, LMWHs are contraindicated in patients with severe renal impairment (creatinine clearance less than 30 mL/min), while UFHs can be used. The risk of HIT during treatment with LMWHs is less than that with UFHs. It is estimated at less than 1%.

4.2 Risk of Oral Bleeding with Injectable Anticoagulants

The risk of post-extraction bleeding is unknown. Little evidence is available for the periprocedural management of injectable anticoagulants in dental extractions. Two approaches are described in the literature; no discontinuation of heparins and discontinuation of heparins prior to the procedure (6–8 h before for UFHs and the day before for LMWHs and resumption depending on the hemostatic control). However, currently there is no consensus regarding whether heparins may be discontinued prior a dental surgery.

5 Conclusion

Oral bleeding may be linked to the use of antithrombotic agents. Drug-induced bleeding may be potentially dangerous during dental surgery. The bleeding risk after dentoalveolar surgery is low and easily controlled by local hemostasis. Perioperative managements of APAs and VKAs are well codified. In contrast, with DOACs and heparins, the optimal periprocedural management remains unclear.

Bibliography

Aframian DJ, Lalla RV, Peterson DE. Management of dental patients taking common hemostasis-altering medications. Oral Surg Oral Med Oral Pathol Oral Radiol Endod. 2007;103(suppl 1):S45.e1–S45.e11.

Ageno W, Gallus AS, Wittkowsky A, Crowther M, Hylek EM, Palareti G, American College of Chest Physicians. Oral anticoagulant therapy: antithrombotic therapy and prevention of thrombosis, 9th Ed: American College of Chest Physicians Evidence-Based Clinical Practice Guidelines. Chest. 2012;141(2 Suppl):e44S88S.

Airoldi F, Colombo A, Morici N. Incidence and predictors of drug-eluting stent thrombosis during and after discontinuation of thienopyridine treatment. Circulation. 2007;116:745–54.

Al-Belasy FA, Amer MZ. Hemostatic effect of nButyl-2 cyanoacrylate (Histoacryl) glue in warfarin treated patients undergoing oral surgery. J Oral Maxillofac Surg. 2003;61:14059.

Alcok RF, Reddel CJ, Pennings GJ, Hillis GS, Curnow JL, Brieger DB. The rebound phenomenon after aspirin cessation: the biochemical evidence. Int J Cardiol. 2014;174:376–8.

Ardekian L, Gaspar R, Peled M, Brener B, Laufer D. Does low-dose aspirin therapy complicate oral surgical procedures? J Am Dent Assoc. 2000;131:331–5.

Bacci C, Maglione M, Favero L, Perini A, Di Lenarda R, Berengo M, Zanon E. Management of dental extraction in patients undergoing anticoagulant treatment. Results from a large, multicentre, prospective, case-control study. Thromb Haemost. 2010;104:972–5.

Bacci C, Berengo M, Favero L, Zanon E. Safety of dental implant surgery in patients undergoing anticoagulation therapy: a prospective casecontrol study. Clin Oral Implants Res. 2011;22:151–6.

Bajkin BV, Todorovic LM. Safety of local anesthesia in dental patients taking oral anticoagulants: is it still controversial? Br J Oral Maxillofac Surg. 2012;50:65–8.

Bajkin BV, Popovic SL, Selakovic SD. Randomized, prospective trial comparing bridging therapy using low-molecular-weight heparin with maintenance of oral anticoagulation during extraction of teeth. J Oral Maxillofac Surg. 2009;67:990–5.

Bajkin BV, Bajkin IA, Petrovic BB. The effects of combined oral anticoagulant-aspirin therapy in patients undergoing tooth extractions: a prospective study. J Am Dent Assoc. 2012;143:771–6.

Bajkin BV, Urosevic IM, Stankov KM, Petrovic BB, Bajkin IA. Dental extractions and risk of bleeding in patients taking single and dual antiplatelet treatment. Br J Oral Maxillofac Surg. 2015;53:29–43.

Blinder D, Manor Y, Martinowitz U, Taicher S, Hashomer T. Dental extractions in patients maintained on continued oral anticoagulant: comparison of local hemostatic modalities. Oral Surg Oral Med Oral Pathol Oral Radiol Endod. 1999;88:137–40.

Blinder D, Manor Y, Martinowitz U, Taicher S. Dental extractions in patients maintained on oral anticoagulant therapy: comparison of INR value with occurrence of postoperative bleeding. Int J Oral Maxillofac Surg. 2001;30:518–21.

Bodner L, Weinstein JM, Baumgarten AK. Efficacy of fibrin sealant in patients on various levels of oral anticoagulant undergoing oral surgery. Oral Surg Oral Med Oral Pathol Oral Radiol Endod. 1998;86:421–4.

Borea G, Montebugnoli L, Capuzzi P, Magelli C. Tranexamic acid as mouthwash in anticoagulant-treated patients undergoing oral surgery. An alternative method to discontinuing anticoagulant therapy. Oral Surg Oral Med Oral Pathol. 1993;75:29–31.

Brennan MT, Valerin MA, Noll JL, Napenas JJ, Kent ML, Fox PC, Saaser HC, Lockhart PB. Aspirin use and post-operative bleeding from dental extractions. J Dent Res. 2008;87(8):740–4.

Broekema F, van Minnen B, Jansma J, Bos RR. Risk of bleeding after dento-alveolar surgery in patients taking anticoagulants. Br J Oral Maxillofac Surg. 2014;52:e15–9.

Cañigral A, Silvestre FJ, Cañigral G, Alós M, Garcia-Herraiz A, Plaza A. Evaluation of bleeding risk and measurement methods in dental patients. Med Oral Patol Oral Cir Bucal. 2010;15:e863 8.

Cannon PD, Dharmar VT. Minor oral surgical procedures in patients on oral anticoagulants- a controlled study. Aust Dent J. 2003;48:115–8.

Carter G, Goss A. Tranexamic acid mouthwash. A prospective randomized study of a 2-day regimen vs 5-day regimen to prevent postoperative bleeding in anticoagulated patients requiring dental extractions. In J Oral Maxillofac Surg. 2003;32:504–7.

Carter G, Goss A, Lloyd J, Tocchetti R. Tranexamic acid mouthwash versus autologous fibrin glue in patients taking warfarin undergoing dental extractions: a randomized prospective clinical study. J Oral Maxillofac Surg. 2003;61:1432–5.

Clemm R, Neukam FW, Rusche B, Bauersachs A, Musazaa S, Schmitt CM. Management of anticoagulated patients in implant therapy. A clinical comparative study. Clin Oral Implants Res. 2016;27(10):1274–82.

Cooke GE, Liu-Sratton Y, Kerketich AK. Effect of platelet antigen polymorphism on platelet inhibition by aspirin, clopidogrel, or their combination. J Am Coll Cardiol. 2006;7:5416.

Davi G, Patrono C. Platelet activation and atherothrombosis. N Engl J Med. 2007;357:2482–94.

Devani P, Lavery KM, Howell CJT. Dental extractions in patients on warfarin: is alteration of anticoagulant regime necessary? Br J Oral Maxillofac Surg. 1998;36:107–11.

Dubois V, Dincq AS, Douxfils J, Iclx B, Samama CM, Dogné JM, Gourdin M, Chatelain B, Mullier F, Lessire S. Perioperative management of patients on direct oral anticoagulants. Thrombosis J. 2017;15:14. https://doi.org/10.1186/s12959-017-0137-1.

Eichhorn W, Burkert J, Vorwig O, Blessmann M, Cahovan G, Zeuch J, Eichhorn M, Heiland M. Bleeding incidence after oral surgery with continued oral anticoagulation. Clin Oral Investig. 2012;16(5):1371–6.

Eikelboom JW, Hirsh J, Spencer FA, Baglin TP, Weitz JI. Antiplatelet drugs: antithrombotic therapy and prevention of thrombosis, 9th ed: American College of Chest Physicians evidence-based clinical practice guidelines. Chest. 2012;141(2 Suppl):e89S–119S.

Evans IL, Sayers MS, Gibbons AJ, Price G, Snooks H, Sugar AW. Can warfarin be continued during dental extraction? Results of a randomized controlled trial. Br J Oral Maxillofac Surg. 2002;40:248–52.

Febbo A, Cheng A, Stein B, Goss A, Sambrook P. Postoperative bleeding following dental extractions in patients anticoagulated with warfarin. J Oral Maxillofac Surg. 2016;74(8):1518–23.

Garnier J, Truchot F, Quero J, Meziere X, Clipet F, Alno N, Frachon X, Delanoue O, Bader G, Lejeune S, Limbour P, De Mello G. 218 tooth extractions in patients tacking platelet aggregation inhibitors. Rev Stomatol Chir Maxillofac. 2007;108:407–10.

Gaspar R, Brenner B, ARdekian L, Peled M, Laufer D. Use of tranexamic acid mouthwash to prevent postoperative bleeding in oral surgery patients on oral anticoagulant medication. Quintessence Int. 1997;28(6):375–9.

Gomez-Moreno G, Aguilar-Salvatierra A, Fernandez-Cejas E, Delgado-Ruiz RA, Markovic A, Clavo-Guirado JL. Dental implant surgery in patients in treatment with the anticoagulant oral rivaroxaban. Clin Oral Implants Res. 2016a;1:1–4.

Gomez-Moreno G, Fernandez-Cejas E, Aguilar-Salvatierra A, de Carlos F, Delgado-Ruiz RA, Clavo-Guirado JL. Dental implant surgery in patients in treatment by dabigatran. Clin Oral Implants Res. 2016b;1:1–5.

Guyat GH, Akl EA, Crowther M, Gutterman DD, Schünemann HJ. Antithrombotic therapy and prevention of thrombosis (9th ed). American College of Chest Physicians. Evidence-based clinical practice guidelines. Chest. 2012;141(Suppl):7S–47S.

Halfpenny W, Fraser JS, Adlam DM. Comparison of 2 hemostatic agents for the prevention of postextraction hemorrhage in patients on anticoagulants. Oral Surg Oral Med Oral Pathol Oral Radiol Endod. 2001;92:257–9.

Hanken H, Gröbe A, Heiland M, Smeets R, Kluwe L, Wikner J, Koehnke R, Al-Dam A, Eichhorn W. Postoperative bleeding risk for oral surgery under continued rivaroxaban anticoagulant therapy. Clin Oral Invest. 2016;20(6):1279–82. https://doi.org/10.1007/s00784-015-1627-9.

Heidbuchel H, Verhamme P, Alings M, Antz M, Hacke W, Oldgren J, Sinnaeve P, Camm AJ, Kirchhof P. European heart rhythm association practical guide on the use of new oral anticoagulants in patients with non-valvular atrial fibrillation. Europace. 2013;15:625–51.

Hughes GJ, Patel PN, Saxena N. Acetaminophen on international normalized ratio in patients receiving warfarin therapy. Pharmacotherapy. 2011;31:591–7.

Karsh ED, Erdogan O, Esen E, Acartürk E. Comparison of the effects of warfarin and heparin on bleeding caused by dental extraction: a clinical study. J Oral Maxillofac Surg. 2011;69:2500–7.

Krishnan B, Shenoy N, Alexander M. Exodontia and antiplatelet therapy. J Oral Maxillofac Surg. 2008;66:2063–6.

Lillis T, Ziakas A, Koskinas K, Tsirlis A, Giannoglou G. Safety of dental extractions during uninterrupted single or dual antiplatelet treatment. Am J Cardiol. 2011;108:964–7.

Madan GA, Madan SG, Madan G, Madan AD. Minor oral surgery without stopping daily lowdose aspirin therapy: a study of 51 patients. J Oral Maxillofac Surg. 2005;65:1262–5.

Mauprivez C, Khonsari RH, Razouk O, Goudot P, Lesclous P, Descroix V. Management of dental extraction in patients undergoing anticoagulant oral direct treatment: a pilot study. Oral Surg Oral Med Oral Pathol Oral Radiol. 2016;122(5):e146–55.

Miclotte I, Vanhaverbeke M, AlubanwoAgbaje J, Legrand P, Vanassche T, Verhamme P, Politis C. Pragmatic approach to manage new oral anticoagulants in patients undergoing dental extractions: a prospective case-control study. Clin Oral Invest. 2017;21(7):2183–8. https://doi.org/10.1007/s00784-016-2010-1.

Morimoto Y, Niwa H, Minematsu K. Hemostatic management of tooth extractions in patients on oral antithrombotic therapy. J Oral Maxillofac Surg. 2008a;66:51–7.

Morimoto Y, Niwa H, Hanatani A, Nakatani T. Hemostatic management during oral surgery in patients with a left-ventricular assist system undergoing high-level anticoagulant therapy: efficacy of low molecular weight heparin. J Oral Maxillofac Surg. 2008b;66:568–71.

Morimoto Y, Niwa H, Minematsu K. Risk factors affecting postoperative hemorrhage after tooth extraction in patients receiving oral antithrombotic therapy. J Oral Maxillofac Surg. 2011;69:1550–6.

Morimoto Y, Niwa H, Minematsu K. Risk factors affecting hemorrhage after tooth extraction in patients undergoing continuous infusion with unfractionated heparin. J Oral Maxillofac Surg. 2012;70:521–6.

Napenas JJ, Hong CH, Brennan MT, Furney SL, Fox PC, Lockhart PB. The frequency of bleeding complications after invasive dental treatment in patients receiving single and dual antiplatelet therapy. J Am Dent Assoc. 2009;140:690–5.

Park MW, Her SH, Kwon JB, Lee JB, Choi MS, Cho JS, et al. Safety of dental extractions in coronary drug-eluting stenting patients without stopping multiple antiplatelet agents. Clin Cardiol. 2012;35:225–30.

Patel JP, Woolcombe SA, Patel RK, Obisesan O, Roberts LN, Bryant C, Arya R. Managing direct oral anticoagulants in patients undergoing dentoalveolar surgery. Br Dent J. 2017;222(4):245–9.

Sacco R, Sacco M, Carpenedo M, Mannucci PM. Oral surgery in patients on oral anticoagulant therapy: a randomized comparison of different intensity targets. Oral Surg Oral Med Oral Pathol Oral Radiol Endod. 2007;104:e18–21.

Salam S, Yusuf H, Milosevic A. Bleeding after dental extractions in patients taking warfarin. Br J Oral Maxillofac Surg. 2007;45:463–6.

Thean D, Alberghini M. Anticoagulant therapy and its impact on dental patients: a review. Aust Dent J. 2016;61:149–56.

Yagyuu T, Kawakawi M, Ueyama Y, Imada M, Kurihara M, Matsusue Y, Imai Y, Yamamoto K, Kirita T. Risk of posextraction bleeding after receiving direct oral anticoagulants or warfarin: a retrospective chort study. BMJ Open. 2017;7:e015952.

Zanon E, Martinelli F, Bacci C, Cordioli G, Girolami A. Safety of dental extraction among consecutive patients on oral anticoagulant treatment managed using a specific dental management protocol. Blood Coagul Fibrinolysis. 2003;14:27–30.

Zeevi I, Rosenfeld E, Avishal G, Gilman L, Nissan J, Chaushu G. Four-year cross-sectional study of bleeding risk in dental patients on direct oral anticoagulants. Quintessence Int. 2017;48(6):503–9.

Drug-Induced Taste Disorders

Vianney Descroix

1 Introduction

Taste is a complex sense inseparable from the sense of smell.

The taste sensation just as the sense of smell is under the dependence of a chemosensory nervous system responding to chemical stimuli by direct ligation to receptors triggering ionic channel opening or second messengers' involvement such as AMPc.

Gustatory information is then driven to the brain stem by different cranial nerves (CN VII, IX and X). Then from the thalamus, signal transmission is transmitted to the primary gustatory area located in the parietal lobe.

Drug-induced taste disorders/modifications are relatively frequent. These troubles can involve three different mechanisms. First, it might be linked with a disturbance in the quality or quantity of saliva which is usually the case with drugs having an anticholinergic effect. The second mechanism is due to a lesion and/or a destruction of the lingual epithelium disrupting the epithelial cells renewal, as it is the case with some antibiotics and anticancer drugs. The last potential mechanism is a modification of the zinc, copper, and vitamin A concentrations. Zinc is essential for the gustin synthesis.

Among the drug-induced taste disorders, dysgeusia is way more frequent than ageusia. Dysgeusia is different of the other taste troubles in the sense that it is a persisting sensation and remains incongruous with expected tastes. A dysgeusia complaint must be distinguished from drug persisting taste or its metabolite accumulation. Dysgeusia can be qualitative, then called parageusia (aliageusia and phantogeusia), or quantitative; hypogeusia, corresponding to a perception threshold decrease and hypergeusia to an increase of this threshold. These quantitative dysgeusia can be either global or selective (salty, sweet, acid, and bitter).

Sometimes, taste disorders arise as an unusual taste, sour, or metallic in mouth.

Such drug-induced disruption, prevalence, and negative impact/incidence are unknown and remain confusing. This results of the involvement of various factors, first the taste disorder tests' heterogeneity, then lack of test allowing the quantitative evaluation of these troubles, also numerous comorbidity factors that can also explain this taste disorder such as the disease itself, and finally the wide variability in the literature concerning drug usage (dose and treatment duration).

Drug-induced taste modifications can be the source of loss of appetite, quality of life alteration, emotional troubles, and obviously drug treatment discontinuity.

V. Descroix (✉)
Université de Paris, APHP, Paris, France
e-mail: vianney.descroix@aphp.fr

© Springer Nature Switzerland AG 2021
S. Cousty, S. Laurencin-Dalicieux (eds.), *Drug-Induced Oral Complications*,
https://doi.org/10.1007/978-3-030-66973-7_8

Table 1 The most commonly responsible drugs for taste disturbances. Adapted from Ackerman, 1997, Doty, 2008, Naik, 2010; Scully 2004

Therapeutic classes	International nonproprietary name
Antianxiety	Alprazolam, buspirone, flurazepam
Antibiotic	Ampicillin, azithromycin, ciprofloxacin, clarithromycin, metronidazole, ofloxacin, sulfamethoxazole, ticarcillin, tetracycline
Antidepressants	Amitriptyline, clomipramine, desipramine, doxepin, imipramine, nortriptyline
Antiepileptic	Carbamazepine, phenytoin, topiramate
Antifungal	Griseofulvin, terbinafine
Antihistaminic	Chlorpheniramine, loratadine, pseudoephedrine
Anti high blood pressure	Acetazolamide, amiodarone, amiloride, amiodarone, bepridil, betaxolol, captopril, diltiazem, enalapril, hydrochlorothiazide, losartan, nifedipine, nisoldipine, nitroglycerin, propafenone, propranolol, spironolactone, tocainide
Anti-inflammatory	Auranofin, beclomethasone, budesonide, colchicine, dexamethasone, flunisolide, fluticasone propionate, gold, penicillamine
Mood regulators	Lithium
Antimigraine	Naratriptan, rizatriptan, sumatriptan
Anticancer	Cisplatin, carboplatin, cyclophosphamide, doxorubicin, fluorouracil, levamisole, methotrexate, tegafur, vincristine
Antiviral	Aciclovir, amantadine, ganciclovir, interferon, pirodavir, oseltamivir, zalcitabine
Synthetic thyroid hormones	Carbimazole, levothyroxine sodium and related compounds, propylthiouracil, thiamazole

Three hundred drugs (Table 1), covering the whole material medica, are potentially responsible for taste disorders.

These disorders arise preferentially with:

- Cardiovascular medications.
- Antithyroid drugs: Carbimazole, propylthiouracil.
- Rheumatoid arthritis treatments: D-penicillamine.
- Antibiotics: Betalactamins, metronidazole.
- Opioid painkillers.

2   Cardiovascular Medications

Almost all cardiovascular medicationsare known as taste disruptors. Among those, adrenergic antagonists, converting enzyme inhibitors, angiotensin II antagonists, calcium channel antagonists, antiarrhythmias, antidiuretic combinations, and coronary vasodilators are included. In fact, more than a third of all the antihypertensive drugs have adverse effects disturbing taste.

2.1   Angiotensin-Converting Enzyme Inhibitor (ACE Inhibitor)

Among all the antihypertensive drugs, ACE inhibitors are those presenting the highest frequency of adverse effects disrupting taste. This implies taste lost, metallic or sugary taste onset, taste disturbance, or imbalance/distortion. This gustatory disruption is increased when ACE inhibitors are associated with calcium channel inhibitors and diuretic drugs.

The principal ACE inhibitor is captopril (Lopril® and its generic drugs). From all the ACE inhibitor drugs, this one is the main responsible of ageusia or dysgeusia complaints. Captopril can modify food tastes from salty to sugary or maintain bitter or salty tastes. These adverse effects are dose dependent when the daily dose is lower or higher than 150 mg/day. Captopril is the only sulfhydryl group containing ACE inhibitor. This fact supposedly explains its highest effects on taste disruption compared to other ACE inhibitors (such as enalapril, for instance). The reason why ACE inhibitors disrupt taste is explained by the zinc chelation, an increase in local concentrations of bradykinins or for yet unidentified mechanisms. Bradykinins act indirectly by increasing prostaglandin synthesis and can finally disturb cellular second messengers.

Effects on taste can be solved spontaneously after a few months of treatment. Most of the time, it is necessary to stop the drug treatment to recover normal taste. However, the dysgeusia might not be reduced or suppressed even after a rapid ACE inhibitor withdrawal.

Finally, each patient and even the same patient can react differently to various ACE inhibitors.

2.2 Angiotensin II Receptor Antagonists

Angiotensin II receptor antagonists (AIIRA)or "sartan" (candesartan, irbesartan, losartan, olmesartan…) are drugs mainly prescribed to treat high blood pressure and heart failure. Losartan (also known as Cozaar®) is probably the most commonly prescribed and has been associated with ageusia and dysgeusia. However, these adverse effects are not linked to blood or salivary zinc concentrations that are normal in "sartan" treated patients.

2.3 Calcium Channel Antagonists

More than half of calcium inhibitors have been reported to be associated with taste disturbance with and without sense of smell disturbance. Drugs containing nifedipine, amlodipine, diltiazem, or bepridil are known to induce dysgeusia.

3 Antithyroid Drugs

It is well known since the early 1950s that thiamazole (Thyrozol®), an antithyroid preparation derived from imidazole and containing sulfur, disturbs gustatory abilities. In the first reported case, the patient lost his/her capacity of sweet, acid, bitter, and salty discrimination just 4 weeks after the beginning of the treatment (40 mg dose).

Three weeks after stopping the treatment, taste ability was back to normal.

Patients with hypothyroidism complain more often of taste disorders than healthy people. Respective roles of thyroid impairment, thyroxin, and other comorbidity factors are not clearly delineated in the taste disorders. Indeed, hypothyroidism patients treated with thyroxin could present better gustatory abilities than healthy people. More precisely, hypothyroidism exacerbates recognition of certain flavors especially bitterness, and thyroxin treatment could restore the threshold back to normal.

Finally, carbimazole (Néo-Mercazole®), also an antithyroid agent, can decrease zincemia and is known to cause ageusia.

4 Anti-Infectious Drugs

4.1 Antibiotics

Although it has been known for a long time that some antibiotics can modify taste, their relative influences on taste and smell senses are rarely empirically demonstrated. Frequent use of antibiotics can trigger other infections such as fungal infections that can themselves be the origin of taste disorders.

Many antibiotics, at the usual salivary concentrations, have by their own acidic, bitter, or metallic tastes and can hence themselves generate a gustatory disturbances.

Metronidazole, for instance, is known for having a metallic taste.

Experimental studies have demonstrated several different antibiotic modifications of sodium, potassium, and/or calcium salts when they are directly applied upon the tongue. In addition, ampicillin decreases the sodium chloride perception.

4.2 Antifungal Drugs

Among those drugs, terbinafine (Lamisil®) is probably the one for which taste disorders are the most documented. Taste loss occurs only few weeks after the treatment starts.

4.3 Antiviral Drugs

As many anti-infectious drugs and antiviral drugs are known to trigger taste disorders and more precisely generate a bitter taste. Protease inhibitors used against HIV and during AIDS are responsible for taste disorders and are known to alter taste perception of other substances. Highly active antiviral treatments are responsible for many taste disorders mainly characterized by an oily after taste. Among the antiviral drugs against the influenza virus, amantadine and oseltamivir are known to be extremely bitter in solution.

Similarly, the very bad taste of aciclovir is known to be responsible for the weak observance of treatment in children for whom tablets need to be crushed given their size for ingestion.

5 Anticancer Drugs

Chemotherapy agents can be particularly aggressive and destroy gustatory and olfactory receptors thus potentially triggering chemosensory disorders. These disorders are usually reversible since it is possible to observe sensory bud regeneration from stem cells once the treatment is stopped. The most incriminated drugs are cisplatin, carboplatin, cyclophosphamide, doxorubicin, fluorouracil, and methotrexate.

Anticancer treatments do not always have a direct action on taste. Most of the time they impair the sense of smell and disturb olfactory mucosae. Besides, immunodepression, caused by certain chemotherapies, can be responsible for fungal pathologies at the oral mucosae level, itself responsible for taste disorders such as dysgeusia.

6 Psychotropic Drugs

6.1 Antidepressants

Many tricyclic antidepressants are associated with taste disorders. They not only have an unpleasant taste but also disrupt other products' tastes such as salt or sugar. The underlying mechanisms are identified at two levels: first, these drugs have strong anticholinergic capabilities responsible for an important mouth dryness and second, they could likely modify membrane sodium, potassium, and calcium channels and impair second messengers directly at the gustatory bud level.

6.2 Antianxiety Agents

Among all the antianxiety drugs, benzodiazepines are the most prescribed drugs. Alprazolam and flurazepam are the two benzodiazepines responsible for dysgeusia development. Benzodiazepines improve taste palatability and can increase the sweetness of certain foods.

7 Conclusion

Many case reports have described drug-induced taste disorders. Such a disturbance can have a real negative effect by deteriorating the patient's quality of life and dramatically reducing treatment observance. Today, there is no prospective study allowing the systematic evaluation of this important adverse effect. In fact, taste disturbance complaints are often multifactorial, and the underlying biological mechanisms are not clearly deciphered.

Oral health professionals should particularly pay attention to the patients' drug treatments in case of taste disturbance complaints.

Bibliography

Ackerman BH, Kasbekar N. Disturbances of taste and smell induced by drugs. Pharmacotherapy. 1997;17(3):482–96.
Bakhtiari S, Sehatpour M, Mortazavi H, Bakhshi M. Orofacial manifestations of adverse drug reactions: a review study. Clujul Med. 2018;91(1):27–36. https://doi.org/10.15386/cjmed-748.
Beutler M, Hartmann K, Kuhn M, et al. Taste disorders and terbinafine [letter]. BMJ. 1993;307:26.
Bong JL, Lucke TW, Evans CD. Persistent impairment of taste resulting from terbinafine. Br J Dermatol. 1998;139(4):747–8.

Deems DA, Doty RL, Settle RG, Moore-Gillon V, Shaman P, Mester AF, Kimmelman CP, Brightman VJ, Snow JB Jr. Smell and taste disorders, a study of 750 patients from the University of Pennsylvania Smell and Taste Center. Arch Otolaryngol Head Neck Surg. 1991;117(5):519–28.

Doty RL, Philip S, Reddy K, Kerr KL. Influences of antihypertensive and antihyperlipidemic drugs on the senses of taste and smell: a review. J Hypertens. 2003;21(10):1805–13.

Hallman BL, Hurst JW. Loss of taste as toxic effect of methimazole (tapazole) therapy; report of three cases. J Am Med Assoc. 1953;152(4):322.

Heeringa M, van Puijenbroek EP. Reversible dysgeusia attributed to losartan [letter]. Ann Intern Med. 1998;129(1):72.

Juhlin L. Loss of taste and terbinafine. Lancet. 1992;339(8807):1483.

Levenson JL, Kennedy K. Dysosmia, dysgeusia, and nifedipine. Ann Intern Med. 1985;102(1):135–6.

Naik BS, Shetty N, Maben EV. Drug-induced taste disorders. Eur J Intern Med. 2010;21(3):240–3.

Schiffman SS, Zervakis J, Westall HL, Graham BG, Metz A, Bennett JL, Heald AE. Effect of antimicrobial and anti-inflammatory medications on the sense of taste. Physiol Behav. 2000;69(4-5):413–24.

Schlienger RG, Saxer M, Haefeli WE. Reversible ageusia associated with losartan [letter]. Lancet. 1996;347(8999):471–2.

Scully C, Bagan JV. Adverse drug reactions in the orofacial region. Crit Rev Oral Biol Med. 2004;15(4):221–39.

Drug-Induced Salivary Gland Disturbances

Sara Laurencin-Dalicieux, Bruno Souche,
and Sarah Cousty

1   Introduction

Drug-induced salivary gland disturbances are the most common adverse effects of drug-related oral manifestations especially in the older, highly medicated, population. Salivary flow reduction has an everyday negative impact on the quality of life and well-being of the patients.

Saliva is an exocrine secretion product that flows into the oral cavity from three pairs of major salivary glands (parotid, submandibular, and sublingual) and minor salivary glands (or accessories glands) disseminated in the oral mucosa. It helps ensure several functions:

S. Laurencin-Dalicieux (✉)
Periodontology Department, Dental Faculty,
Paul Sabatier University, Toulouse, France

Periodontology Department, CHU de Toulouse,
Toulouse, France

CERPOP, UMR INSERM 1295, Paul Sabatier
University, Toulouse, France
e-mail: laurencin.s@chu-toulouse.fr

B. Souche
Toulouse, France

S. Cousty (✉)
Oral Surgery Oral Medecine Department, Dental
Faculty, Paul Sabatier University, Toulouse, France

Oral Surgery Oral Medecine Department, CHU de
Toulouse, Toulouse, France

LAPLACE, UMR CNRS 5213, Paul Sabatier
University, Toulouse, France
e-mail: cousty.s@chu-toulouse.fr

- Food digestion.
- Specific and nonspecific immune defense of the body.
- Phonation.
  Protection against tooth decay.
- Food swallowing.

The secretion is under the parasympathetic (cholinergic) command of the pair of cranial nerves (V, VII, and IX) and sympathetic adrenergic nerves (through the cervical carotid centers upper, middle, and lower centers).

The secretion may vary (depending time and external stimuli) in quality and quantity.

Finally, age is a determining factor in daily salivary flow; xerostomia linked to senescence is a major health problem in institutions for the elderly.

Decreased salivary flow induces caries that can be painless but cause rapid tooth destruction.

Many other elements can trigger or suppress salivation.

Bacterial or viral infections cause hypersalivation, the sight of appetizing food induces the same effect. Conversely, fear causes a quite brutal dry mouth sensation by the secretion of adrenaline.

Drug concentration in saliva can be quite important. For example, it is well known that evidence of the use of illegal psychoactive drugs in a police investigation can be obtained from measuring them in saliva.

S. Cousty, S. Laurencin-Dalicieux (eds.), *Drug-Induced Oral Complications*,
https://doi.org/10.1007/978-3-030-66973-7_9

There is a link between medications and salivation:

- Salivary flow inhibition is the most common drug-related phenomenon.
- Sialagogue effect of some pharmaceuticals is much rarer than the sialoprive effect of medical therapeutics.
- Salivary glands can secrete molecules that degrade medications and as a result produce substances that can alter the physicochemical composition of saliva. This can then cause a taste alterations.
- Sometimes saliva stains can be induced by drugs.

There are lots of drug-induced salivary gland disturbances. These medications impair the patients' quality of life and cause significant morbidity. But no evidence-based lists of these medications exist.

The purpose of this chapter is to help health professionals become aware of interactions between medications and saliva. Oral complications can have adverse effects on patients, such as polycaries and opportunistic infections by alteration of the local immune system. They can also have a systemic repercussion and alter the patients' general health status.

2   Drug-Induced Salivary Gland Hypofunction

As an introduction, we would like to focus on the difference between "salivary gland hypofunction SGH" and "xerostomia."

"Xerostomia" is used to qualify the subjective feeling of dry mouth felt by the patient, even if salivary function is completely normal. Xerostomia is the most common adverse drug reaction affecting the oral cavity. It is more frequent in adults undergoing medication than those without any medication, and middle-aged and older patients are more at risk of xerostomia, due to the fact that they are on multiple medications.

On the other hand, many drugs are able to induce an objective salivary flow reduction (quantifiable drop in salivation, precise dosages of the quantity and/or quality of saliva) due to a "salivary gland hypofunction" or SGH.

Symptoms of dry mouth can vary depending on its severity:

- Sensation of having sticky, dry mouth or throat.
- Thick saliva and shooting.
- Burning sensation in the mouth salivary.
- Dry, cracked lips and tongue.
- Increased thirst.
- Taste changes (cf chapter "drug-induced taste disturbances").
- Difficulty chewing, tasting, or swallowing.
- Speech disorders.
- Problems with his dentures.
- Lesions or infections in the mouth (such as candidosis).
- Cavities.

2.1   Physiopathological Hypotheses

The medications susceptible to induce SGH do not act the same way.

The notion of dose could explain why some patients under the same treatment over a long time could develop a complication such as xerostomia with an increased dose.

Saliva secretion is under the dependence of the ortho and parasympathetic autonomous nervous system. Acetylcholine is the neuromediator enabling the transmission of the message from the neurons toward the salivary glands.

Depending on the salivary glands, the proportion of serous or mucous saliva varies:

- Serous saliva secretion (rich in water) is stimulated by the parasympathetic nervous system.
- Mucous saliva secretion (rich in proteins and more viscous) is stimulated by the ortho sympathetic nervous system.

Drug-related SGH can result from several mechanisms:

- A dysfunction in the nervous control of salivation: sympathomimetic drugs (ephedrine, amphetamines, central antihypertensive), anticholinergic drugs (atropine, antispasmodic, tricyclic antidepressants, antiparkinsonian, antihistaminic, muscle relaxants).

– Direct damage of the salivary glands (anticancer immunotherapies).
– Medication-induced dehydration (increased urine flow with diuretics).

2.2 Drugs Involved

Xerostomia is a very frequent reason for consultations whether it is objective or subjective. We will go through the details of "dry mouth syndrome" patient management further below.

Over 500 drugs are associated with xerostomia. However, few publications in the international scientific literature give quantified evidence of the decrease in salivary flow (that means no difference between subjective and objective xerostomia) and even less of the methods used.

Drugs used for urinary incontinence as well as antipsychotics, antidepressants, anticholinergics, antihypertensives, sedatives, and antihistamines are the main medications known to induce xerostomia or SGH (Table 1).

2.2.1 Drugs Used for Urinary Incontenanace

Recent meta-analyses have shown that drugs prescribed for urinary incontinence are among the major drugs related with xerostomia. Most of them exert their action and thus complications through the antimuscarinic mechanisms. They can be nonselective antimuscarinics (oxybutynin, tolterodine, and fesoterodine) or M3-selective receptor antagonist (darifenacin and solifenacin). Others like mirabegron, a beta-3 adrenergic receptor agonist and alternative to antimuscarinic drugs, seem less likely to cause dry mouth.

2.2.2 Analgesics

Nefopam has a very characteristic atropinic effect thus causing a very embarrassing oral dryness in certain cases. Similarly tramadol in 1–10% of patients (common expected adverse effect) also leads to dry mouth.

Methadone and loperamide (an opioid used as an antidiarrheal drug) have been described as inducers of oral dryness by pharmacovigilance centers.

Finally, cannabis is known to induce an oral dryness.

Paracetamol, which is the basic analgesic for mild to moderate pain, is not described as impairing salivary function.

Lidocaine frequently causes a sensation of dryness of the mouth without it being possible to properly reduce the amount of saliva .

2.2.3 Drugs Used in Cardiology

Antiarrhythmics

Cordarone and dronedarone cause hyposialy (and as a consequence dysgeusia) but these adverse effects remain rare and less than 1% of the treated patients. However, it should be noted that the alteration of the taste is a very subjective notion (cf chapter "Drug-induced taste disruption").

Disopyramide has a clear atropinic effect which causes constipation, disorders of accommodation, and especially dryness of the mouth.

Antihypertensives

Prazosin is the leader of **antihypertensive vasodilator alpha 1 blockers**. They are all able to induce xerostomia.

Central antihypertensives (type clonidine or moxonidine) are also responsible for a xerostomia. However, these "side effects" do not contradict the continuation of the treatment. It is up to the odontologist to implement a clinical follow-up of the dentition of his patient (increase decay risk).

Antihypertensive beta blockers form a very important family in the treatment of high blood pressure. They are also indicated as the background treatment of cluster headache and migraines. They include subclasses according to their short or long half-life, renal or hepatic elimination.

DILTIAZEM calcium channel blockers are prescribed for the prevention of angina pectoris and for the treatment of high blood pressure (hypertension). They belong to the Benzothiazepine family and have as an undesirable effect (rare) the appearance of "dry mouth" sensation. This disadvantage is not observed in other families of calcium inhibitors such as dihydropyridines (Amlodipine, for example).

Table 1 Major medications involved in xerostomia or SGH (according to international literature)

Anatomical main group	Therapeutic subgroup	Chemical subgroup	Chemical substance
Cardiovascular system	Antihypertensives	Imidazoline receptor agonists	Clonidine, moxonidine, prazosin
	Diuretics	Thiazides	Bendroflumethiazide
	Beta-blocking agents	Nonselective beta blocking agents	Timolol
	Calcium channel blockers	Phenylalkylamine derivatives	Verapamil
	Antiarrhythmics	Antiarrhythmics	Disopyramide
Alimentary tract and metabolism	Drugs for functional disorder	Synthetic anticholinergics, quaternary ammonium compounds	Propantheline
		Belladonna alkaloids	Atropine
	Antiemetics and antinauseants		Scopolamine
Genitourinary system and sex hormones	Urologicals	Drugs for urinary frequency and incontinence	Oxybutynin, propiverine, tolterodine, solifenacin, mirabregron, imidafenacin, fesoterodine, darifenacin
Nervous system	Anesthetics	Opioid anesthetics	Fentanyl
	Analgesics	Natural opium alkaloids	Morphine, dihydrocodeine
		Oripavine derivatives	Buprenorphine
		Morphinan derivatives	Butorphanol
		Other opioids	Tramadol
		Other antimigraine preparations	Clonidine
	Antiepileptics		Gabapentin
	AntiParkinson drugs	Dopamine agonists	Rotigotine
	Psycholeptics	Phenothiazines	Chlorpromazine, perphenazine
		Diazepines, oxazepines, thiazepines, oxepines	Loxapine
		Other antipsychotics	Aripiprazole, Paliperidone
		Benzodiazepine-related drugs	Zolpidem
		Other hypnotics and sedatives	Scopolamine
	Psychoanaleptics	Nonselective monoamine reuptake inhibitors	Imipramine, amitriptyline, nortriptyline
		Selective serotonin reuptake inhibitors	Fluoxetine, citalopram, paroxetine, sertraline, escitalopram
		Other antidepressants	Bupropion, reboxetine, duloxetine, vortioxetine
		Centrally acting sympathomimetics	Methylphenidate, dexmethylphenidate, lisdexamfetamine
Antineoplastic and immunomodulating agents	Antineoplastic agents	Monoclonal antibodies	Bevacizumab, nivolumab, pembrolizumab, atezolizumab
Respiratory system	Drugs for obstructive airway diseases	Anticholinergics	Tiotropium
	Antihistamines for systemic use	Aminoalkyl ethers	Doxylamine
Musculoskeletal system	Muscle relaxants		Baclofen, tizanidine, cyclobenzaprine
Sensory organs	Ophthalmologicals	Sympathomimetics in glaucoma therapy	Brimonidine
		Anticholinergics	Atropine

Atropine is used in the treatment of bradycardia. It causes an important hyposialant effect.

As a conclusion, the combination of many drugs used in cardiology can increase the occurrence of adverse effects related to these molecules, such as hyposialia. The administration of these drugs in elderly people may aggravate their oral health.

2.2.4 Antiepileptic Drugs or Anticonvulsants

Benzodiazepines (diazepam, clonazepam), hydantoins (phenytoin) have been suspected of causing xerostomia. In the medical international literature, gingival hypertrophy is well documented in the case of treatment with phenytoin but xerostomy is not.

2.2.5 H1 Antihistamines

Example: cetirizine, hydroxyzine, loratadine, and desloratadine. They all have an anticholinergic effect (dry mouth, constipation, accommodation disorder) that increases with the dose.

2.2.6 Antiemetics

Metopimazine, in high doses, causes a dry mouth sensation. This phenomenon is rare. There is no mention of xerostomia in the family of serotonin (5OH tryptamine) inhibitors, which are Setrons. Metoclopramide is not associated with the appearance of hyposialia.

2.2.7 Antiparkinsonians

The family of anticholinergic antiparkinsonian (biperiden, trihexyphenidyl) are naturally those that most often cause a sensation of dry mouth. This effect is also dose-dependent. More rarely suppurative parotitis has been observed associated with rashes especially in the use of biperiden. Dopaminergic agonists (amantadine, rotigotine, bromocriptine) have been implicated in rare decreases in salivary excretion. Inhibitors of COMT (CATECHOL-O-METHYLTRANSFERASE) including entacapone can induce feelings of dryness in about 4% of patients.

Conversely, it is important to note that LDOPA causes hypersialorrhea. Methyl DOPA used as central antihypertensive has a sympathomimetic action. It can cause a sensation of dry mouth.

Lisuride, a Parkinsonian anti-ergot derivative, also has a depressant effect on salivation. Ergot derivatives of rye (bromocriptine, for example) causes the same sensation of dry mouth.

2.2.8 Antidepressants

The anxiolytics of the family of benzodiazepines (sedative-hypnotics) are not listed as disrupters of saliva.

2.2.9 Anticancer Drugs

Xerostomia is a well-documented side effect of salivary gland radiotherapy, chemotherapy, and graft versus host disease.

In the treatment of cancers of the upper aerodigestive tract, irradiation of the salivary glands (cervicofacial radiotherapy) induces xerostomia with impaired quality of life.

The severity of the involvement of the glands is correlated with the cumulative radiation dose.

Cytotoxic agents cause dry mouth by direct damage to salivary gland.

Differential Diagnosis: Non-drug-Related Xerostomia

There are many other etiologies of xerostomia or SGH. In particular, dysimmune diseases should not be forgotten (Table 2).

Table 2 Differential diagnosis of glandular manifestation

Xerostomia	
Anxiety disorder	
Endogenous depression	
Fibromyalgia	
Bulimia/anorexia	
Status post head/neck radiation	
Systemic disease (sarcoidosis, amyloidosis, hepatitis C virus HCV, human immunodeficiency virus HIV)	
Parotid swelling	
Mainly unilateral	Mainly bilateral
– Acute: Bacterial infection, actinomycosis, mechanical obstruction by salivary duct stones – Chronic: Chronic sialadenitis, neoplasia (pleomorphic adenoma of the parotid gland)	– Acute: Viral infection (mumps, EBV Epstein–Barr virus, CMV cytomegalovirus) – Chronic: Chronic infections (HCV, HIV), diabetes mellitus, alcoholism, anorexia, amyloidosis, IgG4-related disease, hyperlipoproteinemia

Sjögren's syndrome is an autoimmune exocrinopathy. It is a chronic inflammatory autoimmune disease of unknown origin. The diagnosis is based on various criteria.

Current European–American consensus criteria for the classification of primary Sjögren's syndrome:

- Unstimulated salivary flow rate[1] abnormal ≤0.1 mL/min (1 point).
- Abnormal Schirmer's test (<5 mm in 5 min) (1 point).
- Abnormal findings with lissamine green or fluorescein staining (≥5 in Ocular Staining Score or ≥ 4 in Van Bijsterveld Score) (1 point).
- Autoantibody detection: anti-Ro/SSA (3 points).
- Histology[2].
- Focal lymphocytic sialadenitis, Focus score ≥ 1 focus/4 mm², 1 focus = 50 lymphocytes/4 mm² (3 points).

• Diagnosis is considered positive if score ≥ 4 points, after application of inclusion and exclusion criteria.
   - Inclusion criteria: Dryness of eyes and/or mouth for at least 3 months, not explained otherwise (e.g., medications, infection).
   - Exclusion criteria: Status post head/neck radiation, HIV/Aids, sarcoidosis, active infection with hepatitis C virus (PCR replication rate), amyloidosis, graft-versus-host disease, IgG4-related disease.
• The lack of any other potentially associated disease is the key requirement for classification as a pSS.

Management of a Patient Complaining of "Dry Mouth"
1/Clinical Examination.

The aim of clinical examination is differentiate subjective xerostomia from objective xerostomia (SGH). The physician should look for:

Functional signs: Difficulties in swallowing gene, chewing, speaking as well as the frequent need to drink.

Clinical signs: Saliva with whitish deposits, viscous saliva, sticky mucous tissues, absence of salivary film, absence of saliva at the ostium of the main salivary glands (after palpation). Also the presence of oral lesions induced by hyposialia: cervical caries, mucosal atrophy (Table 3) (Figs. 1 and 2).

Additional examinations could be necessary: Quantification of salivary secretion: sugar test, salivary flow measurement at rest and after stimulation.

Finally search for "mouth breathing" and other parafunctions.

Table 3 Major clinical signs of SGH

Salivary signs	Saliva whitish deposits Viscous saliva Absence of salivary film Absence of saliva in the ostium of the main salivary glands (palpation)
Dental signs	Cervical caries
Mucous signs	Sticky mucous tissues Mucosal atrophy in particular in the dorsal face of the tongue: Atrophy, sticky coating blackish brown Multiple mucous injuries (angular stomatitis, …) Exfoliative cheilitis Opportunistic infections: Candidosis, …

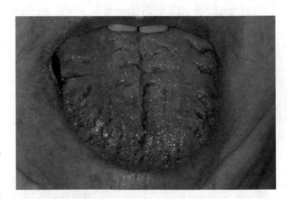

Fig. 1 Fissurated tongue and candidosis in a patient suffering from dry mouth

---

[1]The patient is asked to sit still, not to speak or to chew for 5–15 min; the saliva produced during this time is transferred to a test tube and weighed.

[2]Biopsy: Removal of 3 to 5 labial minor salivary glands from the lower lip under local anesthesiaPCR, polymerase chain reaction.

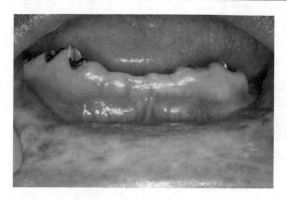

Fig. 2 Rampant decay in dry mouth

2/Medical Interview.

The aim is to define:

- the eventual chronicity of the xerostomia (>3 months),
- the impact on the quality of life and well-being, and,
- the medications that could be related.

3 Other Salivary Side Effects of Drugs

3.1 Drug-Induced Increased Salivary Secretion

Sialorrhea is defined as the increase of saliva amount or flow rate. It is quite uncommon and can occur, for example, during tooth eruption, menstruation, inflammation, gastroesophageal reflux disease. It can also be a symptom of neurologic disease (down syndrome, cerebral palsy, …) or Parkinson.

Local irritation can induce sialorrhea (prosthetic irritation, ill-fitting denture). By the way, it is often difficult to distinguish objective sialorrhea and subjective sialorrhea.

Parasympathomimetic drugs can induce hypersalivation (Table 4).

- Acetylcholine (ACH) increases saliva production: It is a classic parasympathomimetic effect. The synthetic esters of choline (carbachol and bethanechol) also have this effect.

Table 4 Para-sympathomimetic substances increasing the amount of saliva and decreasing salivary viscosity

Direct mechanism	Indirect mechanism
Arecoline	Cisapride
Bethanechol	Neostigmine
Carbachol	Physostigmine
Pilocarpine	Rivastigmine
Muscarine	
Cevimeline	

Choline receptor blocking molecules can be divided into two major groups:

- Muscarinic antagonists (antimuscarinic): The leader of this group is atropine.
  They block muscarinic receptors and are classified in standard terminology from M1 to M5 (M3 receptors are present on glandular cells and smooth muscle cells)
- Nicotinic receptors block the ganglionic transmission of the autonomic nervous system. They are called ganglioplegic. They have limited interest in pharmacology because of their nonselectivity (removal of the target organ). They can cause a wide range of adverse effects but not necessarily hyposialy.
  - Some natural substances like pilocarpine have the same action as ACH. They bind to so-called muscarinic receptors. Muscarinic receptors are located at the neuron–effector junction.
  - Nicotine has a cholinomimetic effect on the ganglion of the autonomic nervous system. These substances have a vasodilating action on the blood system and ensure a greater salivary gland vascularization and thus increase salivary secretion but with a decrease in the salivary rate of the proteins and increase of the aqueous proportion.

Many other drugs are also able to induce hypersalivation: lithium, clozapine, alprazolam, digoxin, and haloperidol, mefenamic acid, theophylline, captopril, nifedipine, and some antibiotic agents (gentamycin, tobramycin, imipenem, and kanamycin).

The management of patients suffering from drug-induced hypersalivation is mainly symp-

Table 5 Saliva and salivary gland involvement

Adverse effect	Xerostomia	Sialorrhea	Salivary gland enlargement
Mechanism	Sympathomimetic effects (anticholinergic) Damage to salivary gland Excreting body liquids (dehydration) Vasoconstriction in salivary glands	Parasympathomimetic effects (cholinergic action)	Hypersensitivity reaction Edema
Clinical findings	Stomatitis, difficulties in eating/speaking/tasting/swallowing, dysgeusia, burning sensation	Drooling	Swelling of salivary glands
Related medication	Anticholinergics, antihistamine, antihypertensive, antidepressant, diuretics	Sympathomimetic drugs	Radioiodine, clozapine, chlorhexidine

tomatic. Anticholinergic agents (such as scopolamine, skin patches for transdermal administration) could reduce the amount of saliva and let the patient stop drooling. Some authors report injection of botulinum into parotid gland.

3.1.1 Discoloration of Saliva

Some medications are known to colorate saliva and other body liquids such as: clofazimine, levodopa, rifampin, and rifabutin.

3.1.2 Salivary Gland Enlargement

Parotid enlargement has been reported as an adverse drug reaction of iodine containing drugs (imaging contrast media). In the treatment of thyroid cancer, radioiodine is frequently used as a therapeutic agent. It can induce salivary gland swelling.

Many other medications cause salivary gland enlargement (Table 5). For example, insulin, methyldopa, phenylbutazone, oxyphenbutazone, potassium chloride, sulfonamide, sodium warfarin, naproxen, guanidine, nitrofurantoin, clonidine, terbinafine, chlorhexidine, doxycycline, diazepam.

amount of saliva, to a true iatrogenic dry syndrome, secondary, resulting in mucositis and the occurrence of multiple decays. This is fully expected in the case of cervicofacial irradiations in the treatment of cancers of the upper aerodigestive tract.

However, in published cases report, methods of studying the amount of saliva emitted are often missed.

The standardization of these tests is perfectible.

There are unquestionably classes of drugs whose ability to reduce salivation is easily recognized: atropine (and derivatives) benzodiazepines belong to these groups.

The practitioner must frequently update the treatment history of his patients to detect any molecule that can induce dry mouth. The imputability of drugs must be evoked in any case of xerostomia or dry mouth.

In addition, the practitioner must of course bring back reports of adverse effects to the regional pharmacovigilance authorities in the face of any effect attributable to treatment.

4   Conclusion

The correlation between xerostomia and drug treatments is well established.

Molecules involved in this phenomenon are multiple. The oral complication can vary from sensation of dry mouth, associated or not with dysgeusia without apparent change in the

Bibliography

Abdollahi M, Radofar M. A review of drug-induced oral reactions. J Contemp Dent Pract. 2003;4:10–31.

Femiano F, Lanza A, Buonaiuto C, Gombos F, Rullo R, Festa V, et al. Oral manifestations of adverse drug reactions: guidelines. J Eur Acad Dermatol Venereol. 2008;22:681–91.

Gil-Montoya JA, Silvestre FJ, Barrios R, Silvestre-Rangil J. Treatment of xerostomia and hyposalivation in the elderly: a systematic review. Med Oral Patol Oral Cir Bucal. 2016;21(3):355–66.

Jayakaran TG. The effect of drugs in the oral cavity - a review. J Pharm Sci Res. 2014;6:89–96.

Porter SR, Scully C, Hegarty AM. An update of the etiology and management of xerostomia. Oral Surg Oral Med Oral Pathol Oral Radiol Endod. 2004;97: 28–46.

Scully C. Drug effects on salivary glands: dry mouth. Oral Dis. 2003;9:165–76.

Scully C, Bagan JV. Adverse drug reactions in the orofacial region. Crit Rev Oral Biol Med. 2004;15: 221–39.

Shetty SR, Bhowmick S, Castelino R, Babu S. Drug induced xerostomia in elderly individuals: an institutional study. Contemp Clin Dent. 2012;3: 173–5.

Shiboski CH, Shiboski SC, Seror R, et al. 2016 American College of Rheumatology/European league against rheumatism classification criteria for primary Sjögren's syndrome: a consensus and data-driven methodology involving three international patient cohorts. Arthritis Rheumatol. 2017;69:35–45.

Stefanski AL, Tomiak C, Pleyer U, Dietrich T, Burmester GR, Dörner T. The diagnosis and treatment of Sjögren's syndrome. Dtsch Arztebl Int. 2017;114:354–61. https://doi.org/10.3238/arztebl.2017.0354.

Sultana N, Sham EM. Xerostomia an overview. Int J Clin Dent. 2011;3:58–61.

Tan ECK, Lexomboon D, Sandborgh-Englund G, Haasum Y, Johnell K. Medications that cause dry mouth as an adverse effect in older people: a systematic review and metaanalysis. J Am Geriatr Soc. 2018;66:76–84. https://doi.org/10.1111/jgs.15151.

Villa A, Abati S. Risk factors and symptoms associated with xerostomia: a cross-sectional study. Aust Dent J. 2011;56:290–5.

Villa A, Wolff A, Narayana N, Dawes C, Aframian DJ, Lynge Pedersen AM, Vissink A, Aliko A, Sia YW, Joshi RK, McGowan R, Jensen SB, Kerr AR, Ekström J, Proctor G. World workshop on oral medicine VI: a systematic review of medication-induced salivary gland dysfunction. Oral Dis. 2016;22(5):365–82.

Vinayak V, Annigeri RG, Patel HA, Mittal S. Adverse affects of drugs on saliva and salivary glands. J Orofac Sci. 2013;5:15–20.

Wolff A, Joshi RK, Ekström J, Aframian D, Pedersen AM, Proctor G, Narayana N, Villa A, Sia YW, Aliko A, McGowan R, Kerr AR, Jensen SB, Vissink A, Dawes C. A guide to medications inducing salivary gland dysfunction, Xerostomia, and subjective Sialorrhea: a systematic review sponsored by the world workshop on oral medicine VI. Drugs R D. 2017;17(1):1–28.

Yuan A, Woo SB. Adverse drug events in the oral cavity. Oral Surg Oral Med Oral Pathol Oral Radiol. 2015;119:35–47.

Zavras AI, Rosenberg GE, Danielson JD, Cartsos VM. Adverse drug and device reactions in the oral cavity. surveillance and reporting J Am Dent Assoc. 2013;144:1014–21.

Drug-Induced Oral Infections

Sylvie Boisramé and Anne-Gaëlle Chaux-Bodard

1 Introduction

Oral infections are among the most common diseases worldwide.

They are numerous and can be induced by commensal microbiotic pathogens. The oral cavity harbors over 700 species of bacteria, virus, fungi, and protozoa. There is a balance between commensal microbiota and oral environmental factors. For example, saliva plays a great role in the oral balance. Oral immunity is both innate and adaptive, with two main mechanisms: cell-mediated immunity and humoral-mediated immunity. The local immune response is modulated by saliva which contains protective proteins.

Sometimes, some of those microorganisms beneficial to our human health can transition from a commensal relationship to one of pathogenicity. On the one hand, the disease-causing bacteria are present in a pathogenic state but oral commensal bacteria more abundant counterbal-

ance their dangerous effect. On the other hand, an environmental modification (inflammation, pH, immunity…) stimulates activity of microbiota resulting in infection or disease.

2 Drugs Leading to Oral Infections (Fig. 1)

2.1 Immunomodulating Drugs

2.1.1 Antineoplastic Drugs

Antineoplastic drugs are used in the treatment of cancer. They are cytotoxic and most of time are myelosuppressive drugs. Some drugs are cell-cycle dependent and some are cell-cycle independent. In this superfamily, there are alkylating drugs (such as busulfan, cisplatin), antimitotic drugs which are natural products derived from plants (such as vincristine, docetaxel, etoposide) or microorganisms (such as bleomycin, doxorubicin), antimetabolites (5-fluorouracil, methotrexate), miscellaneous (rituximab, imatinib mesylate, …), hormones, and antagonists (dexamethasone, tamoxifen, …). Mechanisms of immunomodulation are different, depending on the family they belong to. They also have an indirect immune toxicity through their effect on bone marrow which causes anemia, leukopenia, and neutropenia.

Alkylating agents are able to link with DNA of bone marrow cells and thus have a

S. Boisramé (✉)
Oral Surgery Department, Brest University Hospital Center, Brest, France
e-mail: Sylvie.boisrame@univ-brest.fr

A.-G. Chaux-Bodard
Oral Surgery, Faculty of Dentistry, and Centre Régional de Lutte Contre le Cancer Léon Bérard, University Claude Bernard Lyon I, Villeurbanne, France
e-mail: anne-gaelle.bodard@lyon.unicancer.fr

© Springer Nature Switzerland AG 2021
S. Cousty, S. Laurencin-Dalicieux (eds.), *Drug-Induced Oral Complications*,
https://doi.org/10.1007/978-3-030-66973-7_10

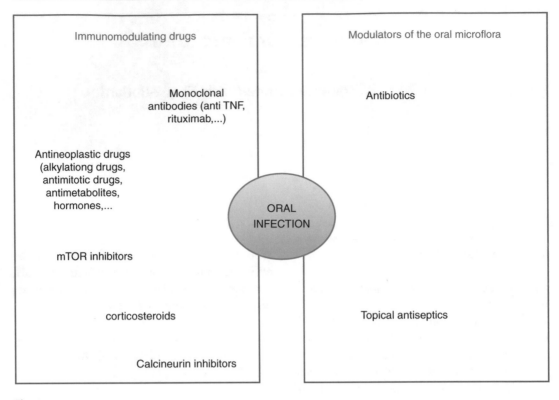

Fig. 1

hematopoietic effect. Topoisomerase inhibitors (doxorubicin, etoposide) inhibit the topoisomerase, which is an enzyme that regulates DNA topology and is essential for the integrity of the genetic material during transcription. The inhibitors stabilize the DNA-cleavable complex and are supposed to have genotoxic effects. Cyclosporin links to purine bases of DNA and thus induces apoptosis and myelosuppression. Antimetabolites block the use of metabolites, through their incorporation in RNA. They are analogs of DNA bases, i.e., 5-fluorouracil mimics pyrimidine.

2.1.2 Other Antimetabolite Drugs

Other antimetabolite drugs such as azathioprine (imidazole derivative of 6-maercaptopurine, also used in renal-transplanted patients), mycophenolate mofetil (used in autoimmune diseases) are also immunomodulators. Azathioprine inhibits the nucleotide synthesis. Its effect is dose dependent. Mycophenolate mofetil is the prodrug of mycophenolic acid which is implicated in the synthesis of guanosine nucleotides. It is able to

induce apoptosis of activated T lymphocytes. Its main mechanism is an inhibition of inosine monophosphate dehydrogenase. It decreases the recruitment of lymphocytes and monocytes and suppresses primary T-lymphocyte response to allogeneic cells and antigens.

2.1.3 Corticosteroids

Corticosteroids are widely used in medicine. They are used in case of inflammatory diseases, autoimmune diseases, cancer, and in long-term administration can lead to immunomodulation. Their mechanism of action is an upregulation of anti-inflammatory proteins. They also downregulate the expression of proinflammatory proteins and have a role in the development and homeostasis of T lymphocytes. They play a role on B-cells through inhibition of NF Kappa B (nuclear factor kappa of activated B-cells). They decrease cell-mediated immunity by inhibiting genes coding for IL 1, 2, 3, 4, 5, 6, and 8. Finally, they are able to cause humoral immune deficiency. Short treatments (inferior to 10 days) are not at risk of increased infection. Medications concerned are prednisone and prednisolone, hydrocortisone, betamethasone, dexamethasone, methylprednisolone.

Topical corticosteroids (creams or sprays) can also facilitate local immunodepression and thus local infection. They are able to pass through the cell membrane and react to a receptor. It then forms a complex which binds to cell DNA, and thus inhibits some proteins like systemic corticosteroids. Oral candidiasis, especially the erythematous variant, which is frequently associated with corticosteroid inhalation in asthmatic patients treated with corticosteroid inhalation. It seems that epithelial lesions favor the penetration of topical drugs.

2.1.4 Calcineurin Inhibitors

Calcineurin inhibitors (CNIs) are a drug family including cyclosporin and tacrolimus. Cyclosporin is a cyclic polypeptide of fungal origin whereas tacrolimus is a macrolide molecule. They have several indications; one of the most frequent is preventing the rejection of organ transplants (kidney, lung, heart, or liver). They are usually associated with adrenal corticosteroids. Cyclosporin is also used in the treatment of graft versus host disease, psoriasis, rheumatoid polyarthritis, dermatitis, etc. They block T-cell proliferation through the dephosphorylation of the cytoplasmic subunit of nuclear factor of activated T cells. It results in the suppression of the generation of pro-inflammatory cytokines. Immunosuppression correlates with the dosage, blood-level, and duration of the treatment.

2.1.5 Monoclonal Antibodies

An international classification of various types of monoclonal antibodies ("mabs") was established and allows distinguishing murine antibodies ("o-mab") from chimeric antibodies ("xi-mab"), humanized antibodies ("zu-mab"), and human monoclonal antibodies ("u-mab").

AntiTNF (tumor necrosis factor) alpha drugs (i.e., etanercept, infliximab, adalimumab, …) are used in rheumatoid polyarthritis, psoriatic rheumatism, or Crohn's disease. They act against both inflammation and innate immunity. The higher prevalence of infection by tuberculosis mycobacteria have been reported in patients with antiTNF alpha treatment. Increased risk of infection from Legionella and Listeria such as other opportunistic infections (also oral pathogens) has been described.

Belatacept is a selective T-cell co-stimulation blocker used in transplantation for prevention of organ rejection. It inhibits T-cell proliferation and production of IL2, 4, IF alpha, and TNF alpha. It increases the susceptibility of opportunistic infections.

Antibodies, anti-leucocyte, anti IL2, IL17 (secukinumab) are used for the treatment of uveitis, ankylosing spondylitis, rheumatoid arthritis, psoriasis. They selectively bind to IL 2 or 17 (17A for secukinumab), which is released by immune cells and thus decrease the cascade of immunity. Basiliximab targets IL2 receptor, rilonacept and canakinumab target IL1, and tocilizumab targets IL6.

Alemtuzumab targets CD52, which is found on normal and malignant leucocytes. It has been approved for the treatment of multiple sclerosis and B cell chronic lymphocytic leukemia.

Rituximab is an anti-CD20 murine/human chimeric monoclonal antibody (which is a pan B cell marker) obtained by genetic engineering. It induces cell death, thus decreasing cell immunity. This monoclonal antibody is indicated in non-Hodgkin's lymphoma, chronic lymphoblastic leukemia, rheumatoid polyarthritis, and granulomatosis.

Brentuximab is used for the treatment of Hodgkin's lymphoma and anaplastic large cell lymphoma. It targets CD30, which is usually often found on diseased cells but rarely on normal cells.

2.1.6 mTOR Inhibitors

mTOR inhibitors (mammalian target of rapamycin inhibitors) are used in oncology (temsirolimus) or in prevention of graft rejection (sirolimus, everolimus). Rapamycin inhibitors bind to an immunophilin and block the cytokine-mediated signal transduction pathways, which leads to an inhibition of T-cell-cycle progression. Their main indications are malignancies (pancreatic tumors, advanced kidney cancer, HER2 negative breast cancer, renal carcinoma, …) and prevention of organ rejection in liver or heart transplantation. Temsirolimus also decreases VEGF expression and lymphocytes.

2.2 Modulators of the Oral Microbiota

Oral mucosal and dental surfaces contain an extremely complex ecosystem of microbial organisms. They live in a delicate balance with each other and with human host. These different species constitute oral microbiota and are in homeostasis with the host immune system. A rupture of this balance causes a dysbiosis which shifts the community leading to disease.

In addition to immunomodulating drugs, other drugs, by modifying the organic component (microorganisms) or inorganic (i.e., pH, salivary flow), are likely to cause this dysbiosis and infection. Antibiotic and antiseptic drugs causing a decrease in salivary flow are particularly concerned.

2.2.1 Antibiotics
Some studies suggest that the competitive balance between microorganisms is altered by antibiotic therapy. Thus, antibiotics that target one kind of bacteria might favor the development of another family of bacteria which was previously contained by the development of the first one. It is particularly acute for oral candidiasis. In fact, a dysbiotic oral microbiome does not ensure important functions such as nutrient supply or protection against pathogens. Moreover, antibiotics interfere with the interaction between the microbiome and the immune system. Some authors report transcriptome and proteome alterations of host tissues. Others highlight the links between antibiotics and immune disorders (like asthma) or celiac disease.

Moreover, they contribute to increase host's susceptibility to pathogens.

2.2.2 Topical Antiseptics
Usual mouth rinses use chlorhexidine gluconate or listerine, which both have an important effect on plaque accumulation and on the overall microbial biomass and its activity. Nonetheless, long-term use of these mouth rinses may induce the emergence of opportunistic oral pathogens.

Decrease in the quality or quantity of saliva leads to a higher risk of developing oral diseases such ascariasis, candidiasis, bacterial infections, aphthous lesions. Indeed, saliva is essential for maintaining oral health. The use of some systemic drugs is the common etiology of xerostomia. Among 500 drugs, more than 42 pharmacological groups have been incriminated in oral dryness.

Antidepressants are the most important drugs inducing xerostomia, mainly tricyclic antidepressants, but selective serotonin reuptake inhibitors (SSRI) combined with benzodiazepines too.

A longitudinal study on elderly reported that chronic intake of diuretics increases nearly six times the incidence of xerostomia.

Other antihypertensives such as beta-blockers or angiotensin-converting enzyme inhibitors have also been reported as xerostomic drugs, producing dry mouth. Some opioids (morphine, codeine, and tramadol), atropine, baclofen, and diphenhydramine can also have an adverse effect on saliva flow.

3 Induced Oral Infections

3.1 Bacterial Infection

Bacterial infection can concern bone of soft tissues. Saprophyte microflora is often implicated in oral bacterial infections, especially in drug-induced oral infections.

3.1.1 Bone Infections
Osteitis is an inflammatory process which can be chronic or acute, localized or diffuse. Its etiology is mainly dental (necrosis) or periodontal (periodontitis or complication of third molar eruption). It can be limited to the cortical bone or periosteum. Chronic osteitis is generally underdiagnosed. The risk is acute during chemotherapy as immunosuppression can induce reactivation of chronic infection. This bone infection is

due to antiresorptive agents and this point is treated in the chapter entitled medication-related osteonecrosis of the jaws.

Alveolar osteitis or dry socket is a complication after dental extraction and is frequently observed in association with contraceptives. The occurrence increases with the estrogen dose in the oral contraceptive. This manifestation can be minimized by carrying out the extractions during days 23–28 of the tablet cycle.

3.1.2 Soft Tissues Infections

Gingivitis: Necrotizing gingivitis is the most frequent infection, especially during chemotherapy. Saprophytic bacteria become pathogens as a result of agranulocytosis. It appears as painful ulcers of the papilla and of the keratinized gingiva. A pseudomembranous layer is often noticeable. Antibiotics must be given to treat these infections. Another clinical presentation of drug-induced gingivitis can also be erythematous and linear, following the collar line.

Periodontitis and especially necrotizing periodontitis can be provoked by the administration of immunosuppressive drugs. Ulcers are associated with gingival bleeding, periodontal disease, pain, halitosis, and submandibular nodes. Antibiotics and surgical treatment are necessary. Necrotizing periodontitis can evolve into an even more severe disease: necrotizing stomatitis, in severe systemically compromised patients.

Actinomycosis is caused by *Actinomyces* spp. and presents like a cervical tumefaction, with poor clinical symptoms. Granulomatous and suppurative oral lesions can be found.

Cellulitis is a polymicrobial infection of fat cells. Its extension is a risk of major morbidity.

Mycobacterium tuberculosis must not be underestimated in chronic immunodepressed patients. Oral manifestations of tuberculosis are rare. The diagnosis is made on an ulcero-vegetant lesion, most of the time located on the dorsal side of the tongue, in a patient with pulmonary tuberculosis and/or immunodepression. The limits of the lesion are thin and irregular with elevated margins and induration. Pain is mostly present. There is no node involvement. The treatment is based on poly-antibiotherapy.

3.2 Fungal Infections

Oral candidiasis is the most frequent opportunist infection. It is usually a locoregional infection but in immunodepressed patients it can be an extensive, systemic infection with potential morbidity. There are various subtypes of Candida but the main one involved in oral candidiasis is *Candida albicans*. It is a saprophyte host of the oral cavity and is present in 30–60% of healthy ambulatory patients. The blastopore stage develops in a hyphal (or mycelial) while becoming pathogenic. Predisposing factors can be diabetes mellitus, malignancy, systemic corticosteroid therapy, and long-term antibiotic therapy. Invasion is possible since candida can bind to keratinocytes and proliferate, thus creating an inflammatory process. Interactions between saliva (especially proteins and immunoglobulins) and levels of candida are important and thus any alteration of saliva flow may induce Candida infection. The patient usually complains of burning mouth and/or metallic taste.

Oral candidiasis infections can occur in cases of oral and perioral infections as:

– Acute variants: Pseudomembranous, erythematous.
– Chronic variants: Hyperplastic, erythematous, pseudomembranous.
– Candida-associated lesions: Sub-overdenture stomatitis, central papillary atrophy, angular cheilitis.
– Keratinized primary lesions superinfected with Candida: Leukoplakia, lupus erythematosus, and lichen planus.

Clinically, oral candidiasis progresses in three steps. First of all, oral mucosa becomes erythematous, and the patient complains of metallic or salted taste. He usually reports burning mouth. After 2 or 3 days, pseudomembranous white spots appear on an erythematous mucosa. The white spots can be removed by friction (Fig. 2).

The most frequent clinical presentation is pseudomembranous, but in a few cases, the

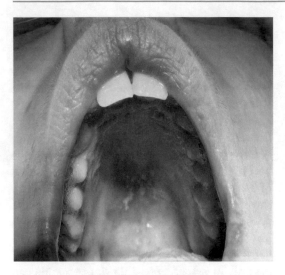

Fig. 2 Pseudomembranous candidiasis with white spots on median hard palate

erythematous stage persists, and the clinical presentation is atrophic and erythematous.

In patients with generalized infections, oral candidiasis infections may be secondary. These lesions are rare and associated with severe immune defects.

Infection usually extends to oropharynx or esophagus.

Atrophic candidiasis is found under removable dentures and presents like erythematous stomatitis, following the contour of the removable denture.

Antifungal treatment (amphotericin, fluconazole, …) must be prescribed. Patients with removable dentures should also be taught to disinfect the prosthesis to avoid reinfection of the oral mucosa, as well as all oral hygiene aids (toothbrush).

Chronic candidiasis is usually localized, and clinical presentations are variable:

– Cheilitis is usually erythematous and presents with a central fissure. The fungal infection is extended thanks the humid conditions in the fissure, mostly due to vertical hypodimension. *Staphylococcus aureus* can also be found.
– Central papillary atrophy concerns the tongue. It presents like an erythematous and atrophic zone, with sometimes the same presentation in the palate.

Diffuse chronic candidiasis presents like white and asymptomatic lesions, which cannot be removed by friction. The last chronic form is hyperkeratotic and is mostly found in the retro-commissural area. In 15% of cases, it can be associated with intraepithelial dysplasia.

Clinical symptoms are poor and antifungal treatment is inefficient.

Other fungal infections can also be found: histoplasmosis, paracoccidioïdomycosis.

Both systemic and topical medications can be involved in the occurrence of candidiasis. Topical or inhalational corticosteroids and overzealous use of mouth rinses can lead to fungal infection. Prolonged use of many drugs (antibiotics, immunosuppressant, and drugs decreasing saliva flow) can induce secondary fungal infection.

3.3 Viral Infections

3.3.1 Cytomegalovirus (CMV)

CMV is a human herpes virus (HHV-5) frequently affecting transplant recipients (almost 60% of these patients). The incidence depends on drug association, with a higher risk for patients treated with an association of alemtuzumab and tacrolimus. The risk decreases when using mTOR inhibitors instead of antimetabolites. The higher risk ratio appears about 100 days after bone marrow transplantation. Oral infections are rare. Clinical symptoms appear in only 25% of the cases. Flu-like syndrome is rare. Oral lesions appear like nonspecific, multiple, pseudomembranous ulcerations with irregular margins. The main risk is a rejection of the graft due to CMV infection. Valaciclovir is preventively instituted in grafted patients. In case of acute CMV infection, ganciclovir must be established.

3.3.2 Human Papilloma Virus (HPV) (Fig. 3)

Human papilloma virus (HPV) is usually associated with immunodepression and may be responsible of most oropharyngeal cancers in non-smokers and non-drinkers patients. It can also induce many benign lesions. More than 150 subtypes of the virus have been identified. The contamination is due to direct contact.

Squamous papilloma is frequently seen in 30–40 years old patients in the soft palate, tongue, lips, or gingiva. It is a benign and exophytic lesion, histologically characterized by para or orthokeratin. The treatment is surgery, with simple surgical blade excision.

Condyloma acuminatum is usually found on the anogenital mucosa but can also concern oral mucosa. This lesion is frequent in the third and fourth decade in sexually active adults, with a high male predilection (19:1). They are pink, sessile, exophytic, and mostly located on the labial mucosa, palate, or lingual frenum. Surgery is also the treatment of choice.

Focal epithelial hyperplasia (FEC), also called Heck disease, commonly affects children and young American Indians and Inuits. Lesions are painless and sessile nodules or papules, with hyperplasia and characteristic mitosoid cells. Lesions spontaneously regress with age but if not, surgery or medical treatment (IF alpha) can be proposed.

HPV is also associated with oral epithelial dysplasia and squamous cell carcinoma (SCC). These lesions are clinically indistinguishable from non-HPV lesions. Their prognosis is better than non-HPV lesions for oropharyngeal SCC but not for oral HPV versus non-HPV lesions.

3.3.3 Epstein Barr Virus (EBV)

EBV is a double-stranded DNA core virus that targets B lymphocytes. Infection may occur in immunodepressed patients and thus, any immunomodulating drug can induce EBV infection. EBV-induced oral infection often occurs in elderly patients or chemo-induced immunodepression (methotrexate, azathioprine, cyclosporine, …). The lesion is often an isolated, indurated, and slowly progressive ulcer and occurs on the tongue, lips, palatal, or buccal mucosa. It can also present as hairy leucoplakia, which is bilateral, elongated, and elevated white lesions of the margins of the tongue. These lesions are asymptomatic. Hairy leukoplakia is often described as a characteristic lesion in HIV patients, and a major marker for immunosuppression. Nonetheless, some authors have described hairy leucoplakia in non-HIV patients such as patients treated with topic corticosteroids. Systemic valacyclovir or local podophyllin resin can be proposed.

3.3.4 Herpes Simplex Virus (HSV) (Fig. 4)

About 60% of adults are chronically infected with HSV 1 and 15% with HSV 2. The virus remains latent in the saliva, and its replication is T-cell dependent. HSV primo-infection or recurrence is frequent during chemotherapy (almost 40% of patients), especially during the most intensive immune suppression period.

Primo-infection can be asymptomatic, but when it is symptomatic, it presents with general symptoms like fever, asthenia, and after a few

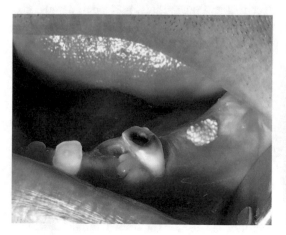

Fig. 3 Wart papilloma on mandibular crest

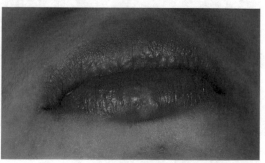

Fig. 4 Human Herpes Simplex virus on bottom lip

days, vesiculous eruption. Vesicles quickly turn into ulcer-like lesions. The lesions heal in a few days.

Recurrence occurs during immunodepression or stress. It begins with virus replication, which is usually non-symptomatic. After a few days, an erythema appears in the area of primo-infection, and then a vesicle. The lesion very quickly turns into a crater-shaped lesion with well-defined margins. Pain is often described. Healing occurs within a few weeks. Acyclovir can be proposed to enhance healing and decrease recurrences. The main risk in immunodepressed patients is severe systemic complications.

Viruses such as herpesviruses have also been known to act synergistically with bacteria in causing diseases.

3.3.5 Varicella-Zoster Virus (VZV)

VZV primo-infection generally occurs during childhood. After a few days of a flu-like syndrome, multiple vesicles appear on the whole body. Oral lesions can also be noticed, but are not systematic. If primo-infection occurs in adults, it can be dangerous, especially in immunodepressed patients in whom it can involve lungs, brain, and liver.

VZV recurrence is localized and is called zona. Its main characteristics are that it appears in a precise nervous area (i.e., the orbitary branch if the trigeminal nerve—V2), it is very painful, and it is unilateral (Fig. 5).

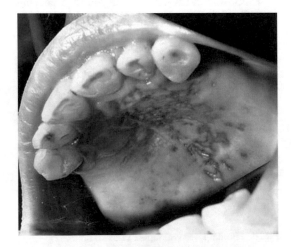

Fig. 5 Zona located on the right side of the hard palate

VZV infection generally occurs weeks after completion of chemotherapy. Lesions generally involve both oral cavity and skin and are painful. The main characteristic is unilateral vesicular lesions. Treatment consists of acyclovir, valacyclovir, or famciclovir.

3.4 Parasitic Infections

Toxoplasmosis is rare and presents as an aphtoid stomatitis. Contamination is due to ingestion of contaminated raw or almost raw meat and exposition to contaminated cat feces. The main risk is for pregnant women, since the parasite provokes major nervous alterations on the fetus.

Leishmaniasis mostly concerns young adults and children. Contamination mostly occurs through a mosquito bite or syringe exchanges. The dog is an important reservoir for the parasite. Lesions can be either cutaneous or muco-cutaneous, but mucosal lesions appear after cutaneous lesions. Mucosal ulcers are usually painless.

3.4.1 Secondary Infections

Fungal, viral, or bacterial infections can be facilitated by oral mucositis. Mucositis is not an infection but this mucosal disease is characterized by ulcerations that disrupt the epithelial barrier. Clinical presentation of oral mucositis varies from erythema to major ulcers, depending on the WHO grade. Its etiology is mainly chemotherapy (such as antimetabolites, alkylating agents, taxanes, anthracyclines, alkaloids…), but also external radiotherapy. Oral mucosa has a high susceptibility for mucositis as its cell turnover is important. Combined with chemo-induced leukopenia, it is responsible for many infections. The most dangerous complication of oral mucositis is probably fungal infection. Disruption of the epithelial barrier facilitates the penetration of microorganisms.

Drug-induced systemic diseases may also lead to secondary immunomodulation and thus increased risk of oral infection. It seems that tacrolimus, used for renal transplantation, increases the risk for developing diabetes mellitus, through its effect on insulin secretion. By the way, it is well known that diabetes mellitus increases the risk of oral infection.

4 Conclusion

This chapter traced in a synthetic way how drugs induce oral infections namely immunomodulating drugs and oral microbiome modulators and also listed different oral infections caused by these drugs.

Bibliography

Abdollahi M, Radfar M. A review of drug-induced oral reactions. J Contemp Dent Pract. 2003;4(1):10–31.

Agbo-Godeau S, Guedj A, Marès S, Goudot P. Xerostomia. Presse Med. 2017;46(3):296–302.

Al Johani KA, Hegarty AM, Porter SR, Fedele S. Calcineurin inhibitors in oral medicine. J Am Acad Dermatol. 2009;61(5):829–40.

Avila M, Ojcius DM, Yilmaz O. The oral microbiota: living with a permanent guest. DNA Cell Biol. 2009;28(8):405–11.

Brode SK, Jamieson FB, Ng R, Campitelli MA, Kwong JC, Paterson JM, Li P, Marchand-Austin A, Bombardier C, Marras TK. Increased risk of mycobacterial infections associated with anti-rheumatic medications. Thorax. 2015;70(7):677–82.

Buffie CG, Jarchum I, Equinda M, Lipuma L, Gobourne A, Viale A, Ubeda C, Xavier J, Pamer EG. Profound alterations of intestinal microbiota following a single dose of clindamycin results in sustained susceptibility to Clostridium difficile-induced colitis. Infect Immun. 2012;80(1):62–73.

Catellani JE, Harvey S, Erickson SH, et al. Effect of oral contraceptive cycle on dry socket (localized alveolar osteitis). J Am Dent Assoc. 1980;101(5):777–80.

Chaveli-Lopez B. Oral toxicity produced by chemotherapy: a systematic review. J Clin Exp Dent. 2014;6(1):e81–90.

De Almeida PV, Gregio AM, Brancher JA, Ignacio SA, Macha- do MA, de Lima AA, et al. Effects of antidepressants and ben- zodiazepines on stimulated salivary flow rate and biochemistry composition of the saliva. Oral Surg Oral Med Oral Pathol Oral Radiol Endod. 2008;106:58–65.

Dongari-Bagtzoglou A. Pathogenesis of mucosal biofilm infections: challenges and progress. Expert Rev Anti-Infect Ther. 2008;6(2):201–8.

D'Souza G, Zhang Y, Merritt S, Gold D, Robbins HA, Buckman V, Gerber J, Eisele DW, Ha P, Califano J, Fakhry C. Patient experience and anxiety during and after treatment for an HPV-related oropharyngeal cancer. Oral Oncol. 2016;60:90–5.

Feller L, Khammissa RA, Chandran R, Altini M, Lemmer J. Oral candidosis in relation to oral immunity. J Oral Pathol Med. 2014;43(8):563–9. https://doi.org/10.1111/jop.12120; Epub 2013 Oct 9

Ghaffar F, Muniz LS, Katz K, Smith JL, Shouse T, Davis P, McCracken GH Jr. Effects of large dosages of amoxicillin/clavulanate or azithromycin on nasopharyngeal carriage of Streptococcus pneumoniae, Haemophilusinfluenzae, nonpneumococcal alpha-hemolytic streptococci, and Staphylococcus aureus in children with acute otitis media. Clin Infect Dis. 2002;34(10):1301–9.

Guarner F, Malagelada J-R. Gut flora in health and disease. Lancet. 2003;361:512–9.

Habbab KM, Moles DR, Porter SR. Potential oral manifestations of cardiovascular drugs. Oral Dis. 2010;16(8):769–73.

Katabathina V, Menias CO, Pickhardt P, Lubner M, Prasad SR. Complications of immunosuppressive therapy in solid organ transplantation. Radiol Clin N Am. 2016;54(2):303–19.

Langdon A, Crook N, Dantas G. The effects of antibiotics on the microbiome throughout development and alternative approaches for therapeutic modulation. Genome Med. 2016;8(1):39.

Lichtman JS, Ferreyra JA, Ng KM, Smits SA, Sonnenburg JL, Elias JE. Host-microbiota interactions in the pathogenesis of antibiotic-associated diseases. Cell Rep. 2016;14(5):1049–61.

Marild K, Ye W, Lebwohl B, Green PH, Blaser MJ, Card T, Ludvigsson JF. Antibiotic exposure and the development of coeliac disease: a nationwide case-control study. BMC Gastroenterol. 2013;13:109.

Murray Thomson W, Chalmers JM, John Spencer A, Slade GD, Carter KD. A longitudinal study of medication exposure and xerostomia among older people. Gerodontology. 2006;23:205–13.

Muzyka BC. Oral fungal infections. Dent Clin N Am. 2005;49(1):49–65, viii

Papapanou PN, Sanz M, et al. Periodontitis: consensus report of workgroup 2 of the 2017 world workshop on the classification of periodontal and Peri-implant diseases and conditions. J Periodontol. 2018;89(Suppl 1):S173–82.

Patil S, Rao RS, Majumdar B, Anil S. Clinical appearance of oral Candida infection and therapeutic strategies. Front Microbiol. 2015;6:1391.

Prasal JL, Bilodeau EA. Oral hairy leukoplakia in patients without HIV: presentation of 2 new cases. Oral Surg Oral Med Oral Pathol Oral Radiol. 2014;118(5):e151–60.

Roduit C, Scholtens S, de Jongste JC, Wijga AH, Gerritsen J, Postma DS, Brunekreef B, Hoekstra MO, Aalberse R, Smit HA. Asthma at 8 years of age in children born by caesarean section. Thorax. 2009;64(2):107–13.

Salvatori O, Puri S, Tati S, Edgerton MJ. Innate immunity and saliva in Candida albicans-mediated Oral diseases. Dent Res. 2016;95(4):365–71.

Samaranayake LP. Superficial oral fungal infections. Curr Opin Dent. 1991;1(4):415–22.

Scheen AJ. International classification of various types of monoclonal antibodies. Rev Med Liege. 2009;64(5–6):244–7.

Scully C, Bagan JV. Adverse drug reactions in the orofacial region. Crit Rev Oral Biol Med. 2004;15:221–39.

Slots J. Herpesviral-bacterial synergy in the pathogenesis of human periodontitis. Curr Opin Infect Dis. 2007;20(3):278–83.

Sreebny LM. Saliva in health and disease: an appraisal and update. Int Dent J. 2000;50(3):140–61.

Stojanov IJ, Woo SB. Human papillomavirus and Epstein-Barr virus associated conditions of the oral mucosa. Semin Diagn Pathol. 2015;32(1):3–11.

Terai H, Shimahara M. Atrophic tongue associated with Candida. Oral Pathol Med. 2005;34(7):397–400.

Walker CB. Microbiological effects of mouthrinses containing antimicrobials. J Clin Periodontol. 1988;15(8):499–505.

Wiseman AC. Immunosuppressive Medications. Clin J Am Soc Nephrol. 2016;11(2):332–43.

Wong HM. Oral complications and management strategies for patients undergoing cancer therapy. Sci World J. 2014;2014:581795.

Wu YM, Yan J, Ojcius DM, Chen LL, Gu ZY, Pan JP. Correlation between infections with different genotypes of human cytomegalovirus and Epstein-Barr virus in subgingival samples and periodontal status of patients. J Clin Microbiol. 2007;45(11):3665–70.

Drug-Induced Facial Diseases

Marie Masson and Carle Paul

1 Introduction

When considering drug-induced oral complications, it is difficult not to take into consideration the perioral and the facial medication-related manifestations. This chapter describes the main facial dermatosis which can be related to various drugs based on a list of drugs reported in the literature.

The following facial dermatitis have been treated:

- Acneiform eruption.
- Rosacea—perioral dermatitis.
- Seborrheic dermatitis.
- Psoriasis.
- Photosensitivity.
- Subacute cutaneous lupus, lupus erythematosus tumidus, cutaneous chronic lupus erythematous.
- Hypertrichosis—trichomegaly.
- Cheilitis.
- Angioedema.
- Acute localized exanthematous pustulosis.

The list of causal drugs is presented in a glossary classified by therapeutic class and alphabetic order at the end of this chapter.

M. Masson · C. Paul (✉)
Department of Dermatology, Larrey Hospital, CHU de Toulouse, Toulouse, France
e-mail: paul.c@chu-toulouse.fr

2 Acneiform Eruption

Acne is a common skin condition that affects adolescents and young adults. Drug-induced acne is a condition associated with certain medications. It may affect individuals of any age group.

2.1 Clinical Presentation

Clinical presentation is characterized by erythematous or pustular lesions on the face, neck, shoulders, and other regions (Fig. 1).

2.2 Drug-Induced Acne-like Eruption

The main drugs reported responsible for acneiform eruption are:

- **Antimicrobial drugs**: Isoniazid (antituberculosis drugs)(+++).
- **Hormonal drugs**: Anabolic steroids(+++), testosterone(+++), androgens (oral contraceptives, injections, and progesterone implants).
- **Immunosuppressive drugs**: Corticosteroids (intra nasal, inhaled, or systemic)(+++), cyclosporine(++), sirolimus, lenalidomide.
- **Anticancer drugs**: Epidermal growth factor receptor inhibitors (erlotinib, gefitinib,

© Springer Nature Switzerland AG 2021
S. Cousty, S. Laurencin-Dalicieux (eds.), *Drug-Induced Oral Complications*,
https://doi.org/10.1007/978-3-030-66973-7_11

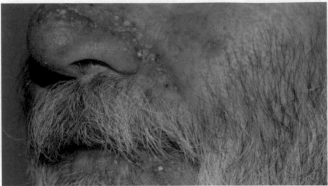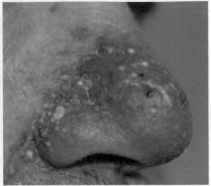

Fig. 1 Acneiform eruption

cetuximab, bevacizumab) **(+++)**, tyrosine kinase inhibitor (sorafenib, imatinib).
- **Antipsychotic or anticonvulsant drugs:** Lithium**(+++)**, sertraline, escitalopram, trazodone, haloperidol, aripiprazole, amineptine, phenytoin **(++)**, carbamazepine, sodium valproate.
- **Vitamin**: Vitamin B6 and 12.
- **Others***: Medications containing halogens.

Few cases have been reported with: *Azathioprine, tumor necrosis factor-alpha inhibitors, quinidine, danazol.*

2.3 Management

For drug-induced rosacea-like dermatitis, discontinuation of the drug is mandatory. Topical treatment with benzoyl peroxide, topical retinoids can be used. Severe disease may require oral tetracyclines.

3 Rosacea and Perioral Dermatitis

Rosacea is a common, chronic cutaneous disorder with a prevalence of 0.5–10%, predominantly affecting women. Factors that exacerbate the disease include genetic predisposition as well as external factors such as exposure to UV light, high temperature, and diet.

3.1 Clinical Presentation

The disease presents with transient flushing, persistent facial redness, telangiectasias, and the presence of centrofacial inflammatory papules and pustules (Figs. 2 and 3).

3.2 Drug-Induced Rosacea-like Eruption

These agents include:

- **Immunosuppressive drugs**: Topical immunomodulators (tacrolimus, pimecrolimus) **(+++)**, topical, nasal, or systemic steroids**(+++)**, etanercept.
- **Anticancer drugs**: Epidermal growth factor receptor inhibitors **(+++)** (erlotinib, gefitinib, cetuximab, lapatinib), 5-fluorouracil, nivolumab, ipilimumab.
- **Others: Preservatives**: Oral parabens. **Vitamin**: vitamin B complex **(+++)**, pyridoxine **(+++)**.
- **Cardiovascular drugs**: Calcium channel blockers, selective phosphodiesterase 5 inhibitors.
- **Immunomodulator drugs**: Interferon alpha.
- **Antiviral drugs:** Ribavirin.

Isolated cases of perioral dermatitis have been reported after:

- **Dental cares:** High fluoride dentifrice.

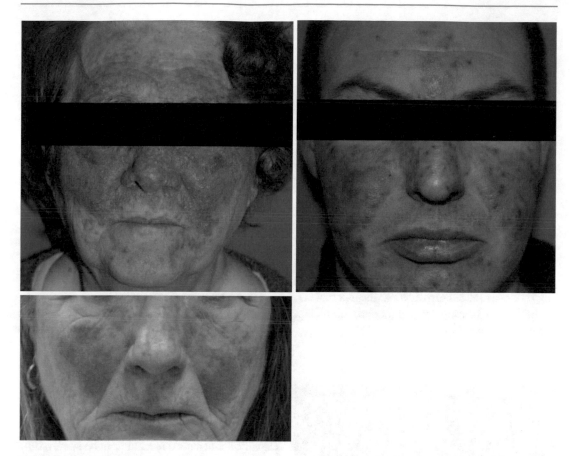

Fig. 2 Rosacea-like dermatitis

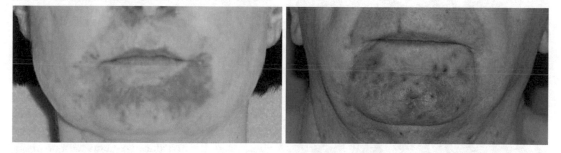

Fig. 3 Perioral dermatitis

3.3 Management

Classical treatment of rosacea may be prescribed. This includes topical metronidazole or topical ivermectin alone or in combination with oral tetracyclines.

4 Seborrheic Dermatitis-like Eruption

Seborrheic dermatitis is a chronic dermatosis most frequently affecting males with a predilection on seborrheic areas. Although the exact pathogenesis remains unknown *Malassezia* yeasts, hormones (androgens), sebum levels, and immune response have been considered to play a role. Other factors including drugs, temperatures, and stress may exacerbate seborrheic dermatitis.

Seborrheic dermatitis has also been associated with diseases such as HIV infection, ORL cancers, or neurologic disorders particularly Parkinson's disease.

4.1 Clinical Presentation

Seborrheic dermatitis is characterized by erythematous patches or plaques with scaling affecting the so-called seborrheic area: the external ear, glabella, hair-bearing areas of the face, nasolabial folds, and scalp (Fig. 4).

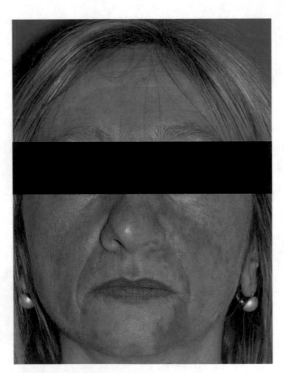

Fig. 4 Seborrheic dermatitis

4.2 Drug-Induced Seborrheic Dermatitis-like Eruption

Anecdotal reports include:

- **Anticancer drugs:** Epidermal growth factor receptor inhibitors (+++)(dasatinib, erlotinib, gefitinib, sorafenib, sunitinib, cetuximab, erlotinib), interleukin 2, topical or systemic 5-fluorouricil, dabrafenib, vemurafenib, and trametinib.
- **Cardiovascular drugs:** Methyldopa.
- **Immunomodulator drugs:** Interferon alpha.
- **Antifungal drugs**: Griseofulvin.
- **Antimicrobial drugs**: Ethionamide.
- **Vitamin A derivative**: Isotretinoin.
- **H2 antagonist**: Cimetidine.
- **Antipsychotic or neuroleptic agents**: Haloperidol, lithium, chlorpromazine, buspirone, phenothiazine, thiothixene.
- **Others**: Gold, methoxsalen, psoralens.

4.3 Management

Usually, seborrheic dermatitis can be successfully treated with topical application of ketoconazole 2% shampoo for the scalp and face twice a week or with the use of antifungal creams (ciclopirox).

5 Psoriasis

Psoriasis is a common chronic inflammatory skin disease affecting 1–3% of population. In some people, psoriasis is drug-induced or drug-aggravated. It can occur in patients with no previous history of psoriasis.

5.1 Clinical Presentation

Lesions are characterized by symmetrically distributed, well-defined scaly plaques (Fig. 5).

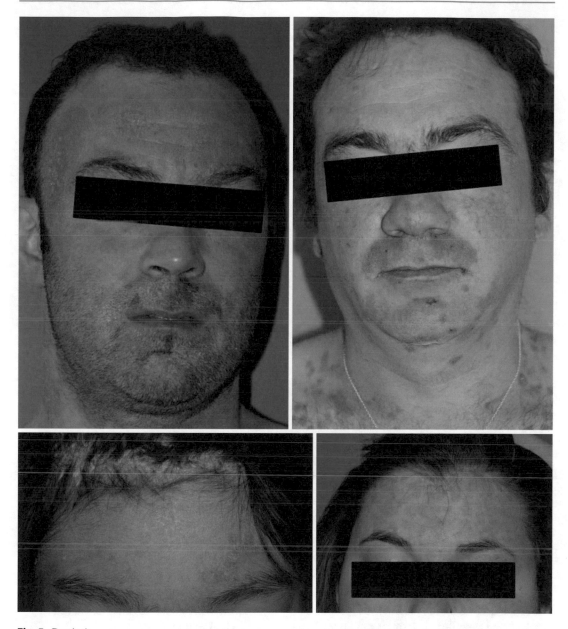

Fig. 5 Psoriasis

5.2 Drug-Induced Psoriasis

The most commonly reported drugs are:

– **Cardiovascular drugs**: β-blockers(+++).
– **Antipsychotic drugs**: Lithium(+++).
– **Antimalarial drugs**: Hydroxychloroquine, chloroquine(+++).

– **Nonsteroidal anti-inflammatory drugs (NSAIDs)(+++):** Indomethacin, phenylbutazone, ibuprofen, meclofenamate, naproxen.

Anecdotal reports include:

– **Cardiovascular drugs**: Angiotensin-converting enzyme inhibitors (++) (captopril, enalapril, ramipril) chlorthalidone, digoxin, clonidine, amiodarone, quinidine, calcium channel blockers.

– **Lipid-lowering drug:** Gemfibrozil (++).
– **Antimicrobial drugs**: Tetracyclines (++), macrolides and penicillin and penicillin derivated, cotrimoxazole.
– **H2 antagonist**: Cimetidine.
– **Hormonal drugs**: Testosterone/estrogens.
– **Immunomodulator drugs**: Interferons (++), imiquimod.
– **Antifungal medications**: Terbinafine (++).
– **Anticonvulsant drugs:** Levetiracetam, sodium valproate, acetazolamide, and carbamazepine.
– **Antipsychotic or neuroleptic drugs**: Fluoxetine, venlafaxine, benzodiazepines, neuroleptic (olanzapine).
– **Immunosuppressive drugs**: Tumor necrosis factor-alpha (TNF-alpha) inhibitors (infliximab, adalimumab, etanercept) (++), withdrawal from systemic steroids, cyclosporine (−).
– **Oral antidiabetic drugs**: Metformin, glibenclamide.
– **Anticancer drugs**: Pegylated-liposomal doxorubicin, mitomycin, nivolumab, rituximab, sorafenib, imatinib.
– **Others**: Icodextrin, botulinum A toxin, recombinant granulocyte-macrophage colony stimulating factors.

5.3   Management

In drug-induced psoriasis, discontinuation of the offending drug must be weighed against the benefit of the drug. In some patients, maintenance of the drug and specific psoriasis treatment might be the best option. The psoriasis treatment algorithm should mirror the one of psoriasis vulgaris.

---

6   Photosensitivity, Phototoxicity, and Photoallergic Reactions

Drug-induced photosensitivity refers to the development of skin lesions on sun-exposed areas due to concomitant exposure to a chemical agent and sunlight.

6.1   Clinical Presentation

Erythema associated with pruritus, burning or pain in sun-exposure area. Upper eyelid, sub-chin triangle, retro-auricular spaces are usually respected (Fig. 6).

6.2   Drug-Induced Photosensitivity

Topical drugs (photoallergic reaction or phototoxic reaction):

– **Nonsteroidal anti-inflammatory drugs (NSAIDs):** Benzylamine, piroxicam, diclofenac, ketoprofen.
– **Others**: Acyclovir, dibucaine, hydrocortisone, fenofibrate, halogenated salicylanilides, chlorpromazine, coal tar, benzoyl peroxide, benzocaine, erythromycin.

Systemic drugs (photoallergic reaction or phototoxic reaction):

– **Antimicrobials drugs**: Tetracyclines, fluoroquinolones third-generation cephalosporins, antituberculosis medications (isoniazid, pyrazinamide), sulfonamides derivates.
– **Antimalarial drugs:** Quinine.
– **Antifungal drugs:** Voriconazole, itraconazole, ketoconazole, griseofulvin, fluconazole.
– **Antiviral drugs:** Efavirenz.
– **Nonsteroidal anti-inflammatory drugs (NSAIDs)**
– **Cardiovascular drugs:** Diuretics: Hydrochlorothiazide, indapamide, furosemide, triamterene. Angiotensin-converting enzyme inhibitors: Captopril, ramipril, enalapril, valsartan, quinapril. Calcium channel blockers: Amlodipine, nifedipine, diltiazem. Others: Tilisolol, rilmenidine, methyldopa. Antiarrhythmics: Amiodarone.

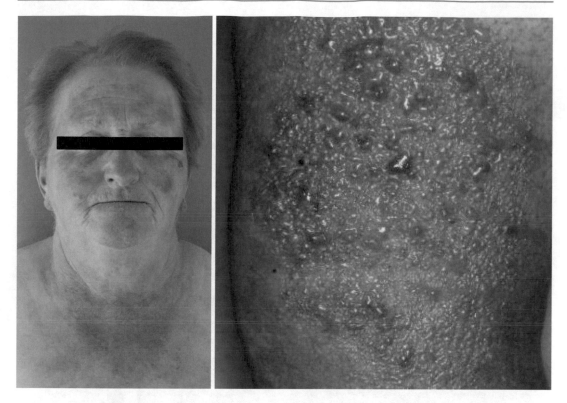

Fig. 6 Drug-induced photosensitivity

- **Lipid-lowering drugs:** Simvastatin, atorvastatin, pravastatin, fenofibrate.
- **Psychotics or neuroleptics drugs:** Chlorpromazine, thioridazine, fluphenazine, trifluoperazine, perphenazine, perazine, olanzapine, clozapine, protriptyline, amitriptyline, imipramine, desipramine, clomipramine, escitalopram, citalopram, paroxetine, fluvoxamine, fluoxetine, sertraline, venlafaxine, phenelzine, alprazolam, chlordiazepoxide.
- **Anticancer drugs:** Vandetanib, imatinib, 5-fluorouracil, capecitabine, paclitaxel, hydroxyurea, dacarbazine, vinblastine, epirubicin, vemurafenib.

6.3 Management

Management is based on sun protection measures which can be enhanced with therapeutic education by trained nurses. Appropriate sun avoidance, the use of clothes filtering UV light, and the use of high sun protection factor sunscreens are recommended.

7 Subacute Cutaneous Lupus Erythematosus (SCLE), Chronic Cutaneous Lupus Erythematosus (CCLE), and Lupus Erythematosus Tumidus (LET)

Drug-induced lupus erythematosus is a lupus-like syndrome related to drug exposure (from 1 month to as long as over a decade) which resolves after discontinuation of the drug.

7.1 Clinical Presentation (Fig. 7)

SCLE is generally typical photosensitive, symmetric, nonscarring annular polycyclic, or papulosquamous lesions usually on sun-exposed area.

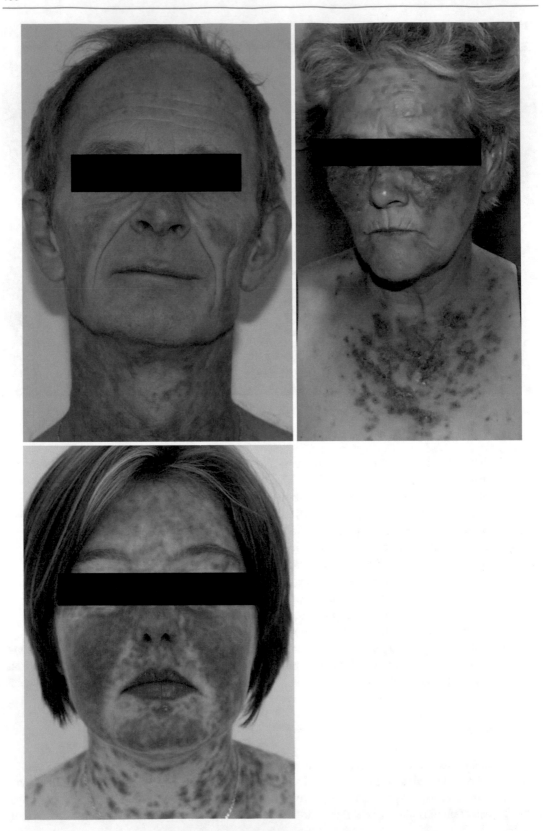

Fig. 7 Drug-induced lupus erythematosus

CCLE are red, inflamed patch with scales and crusts. The center areas may appear lighter in color with an atrophic aspect.

LET is characterized by single or multiple erythematous or violaceous indurated, urticarial plaques with smooth, non-scaling surface.

7.2 Drug-Induced Cutaneous Lupus

For SCLE, the most commonly implicated drugs are: **proton pump inhibitors (PPIs), thiazide diuretics, angiotensin-converting enzyme inhibitors, calcium channel blockers, anticancer, and antifungals drugs.**

All drugs that have been associated with drug-induced SCLE are listed below:

- **Proton pump inhibitor**: Lansoprazole, pantoprazole, omeprazole (+++).
- **Cardiovascular drugs:**
  - Aspirin, ticlopidine.
  - Thiazides (+++): Hydrochlorothiazide +/− triamterene, chlorothiazides.
  - Angiotensin-converting enzyme inhibitors (+++): Captopril, cilazapril, enalapril, lisinopril.
  - β-blockers,
  - Calcium channel blockers (+++): Diltiazem, nifedipine, nitrendipine, verapamil, cinnarizine.
  - Aldactone.
- **Lipid-lowering drugs**: Statins: Pravastatin, simvastatin (+++).
- **Antifungal drugs**: Terbinafine (+++), griseofulvin.
- **Immunosuppressive agents**: Tumor necrosis factor-alpha antagonists (etanercept, infliximab, adalimumab), efalizumab, methotrexate, leflunomide.

- **Immunomodulatory agents**: Interferon alpha and beta.
- **Anticancer agents (+++)**: Adriamycin, 5-fluoroouracil, tamoxifen, docetaxel, paclitaxel, col. 3, leuprorelin.
- **Anticonvulsant agent**: Phenytoin, carbamazepine (+++).
- **NSAIDS**: Naproxen, piroxicam, celecoxib.
- **Antipsychotic or neuroleptic drugs**: Thiethylperazine, benzodiazepines (+++).
- **H2 antagonist**: Ranitidine (anti H2).
- **Hormonal drugs**: Thyroid medications.
- **Others**: Tiotropium, bupropion.

For CCLE, fluorouracil agents and NSAID have been reported as possible implicated drugs. Isolated cases have been triggered by pantoprazole and anti-TNFα agents.

For LET, rare cases have been attributed to anti-TNFα agents (infliximab and adalimumab), ustekinumab, angiotensin-converting enzyme inhibitors, and bortezomib, a proteasome inhibitor used for the treatment of multiple myeloma.

8 Hypertrichosis

Hirsutism is excessive body hair in men and women on parts of the body where hair is normally absent or minimal, such as on the chin or chest in particular, or the face or body in general. The cause is mainly hyperandrogenism, which may be of ovarian or adrenal origin. It may be part of a rare metabolic syndrome, drug induced, or idiopathic.

8.1 Clinical Presentation

Excessive amounts of dark, course hair on body areas where men typically grow hair—face, chest, and back (Fig. 8).

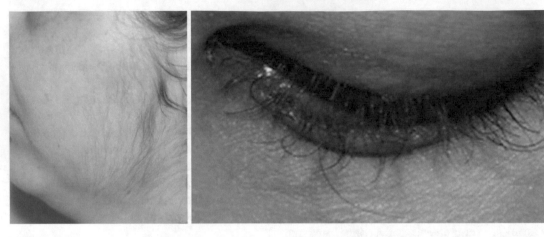

Fig. 8 Hirsutism

8.2 Drug-Induced Hirsutism

The use of the following drugs has been associated with hirsutism/excessive hair growth:

- **Cardiovascular drugs**: Methyldopa (Aldomet).
- **Antipsychotics or Neuroleptics drugs:** Phenothiazines, phenytoin, metoclopramide, reserpine (Serpasil).
- **Immunosuppressive drugs:** Cyclosporine, corticosteroids.
- **Hormonal drugs**: Danazol (Danocrine), anabolic steroids, progestins, testosterone, oral contraceptives (OCs) that contain levonorgestrel, norethindrone, and norgestrel induce more powerful androgen activity, while those that include ethynodiol diacetate, norgestimate, and desogestrel have lesser androgenic activity, Norplant.

Drugs that also result in hyperprolactinemia can cause hirsutism.

8.3 Drug-Induced Trichomegaly

- **Anticancer drugs:** Epidermal growth factor receptor inhibitors (erlotinib, cetuximab), gefitinib.

- **Prostaglandin analogue:** Bimatoprost, latanoprost.
- **Immunosuppressive drugs:** Topical steroid, cyclosporine.
- **Immunomodulator drugs:** Interferon.
- **Others**: Minoxidil, iodine.

8.4 Management

When it is possible, the drug suspected should be stopped. When drug interruption is impossible, laser hair removal and electrolysis can be helpful.

9 Cheilitis

Cheilitis is an inflammation of the lips. It may be acute or chronic, touch the skin part and/or the vermilion of both lips.

9.1 Clinical Presentation

Erythematous-squamous or erosive lesions of the lips which may include the perioral skin (skin around the mouth), the vermilion border, or the labial mucosa (Fig. 9).

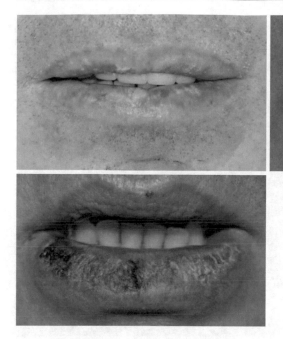

Fig. 9 Cheilitis

9.2 Drug-Induced Cheilitis

This adverse event is commonly observed with:

- **Vitamin A derivative:** Isotretinoin or acitretin (+++).
- **Antiretroviral drug**: Indinavir (+++).
- **Anticancer agents:** Tyrosine kinase inhibitor–targeted agent as sorafenib; the cheilitis is frequently associated with hand-foot skin reaction.
- **Others**: Methamphetamine and heroin users may show xerotic cheilitis. Hallucinogens can induce xerostomia, which predisposes patients to angular cheilitis.

10 Angioedema

Angioedema can be associated with several drugs. There are two basic mechanisms of angioedema formation. The first mechanism is histamine related and this type of angioedema is responsive to oral steroids and antihistamines. This represents the most common form of angioedema. More rarely, angioedema may be related to bradykinin. They do not respond to antihistamine and oral steroids. The most frequent culprit rug for bradykinin-related angioedema is angiotensin-converting enzyme inhibitors.

10.1 Clinical Presentation

It manifests as a swelling of the face, lips, or tongue with or without urticaria (Fig. 10).

10.2 Drug-Induced Nonallergic and Isolated Angioedema

Bradykinin-mediated angioedema is not associated with pruritus or urticaria.

10.3 Angioedema Have Been Reported with

- **Cardiovascular drugs**: IEC (captopril, enalapril, lisinopril) **(+++)**, ARAII (candesartan,

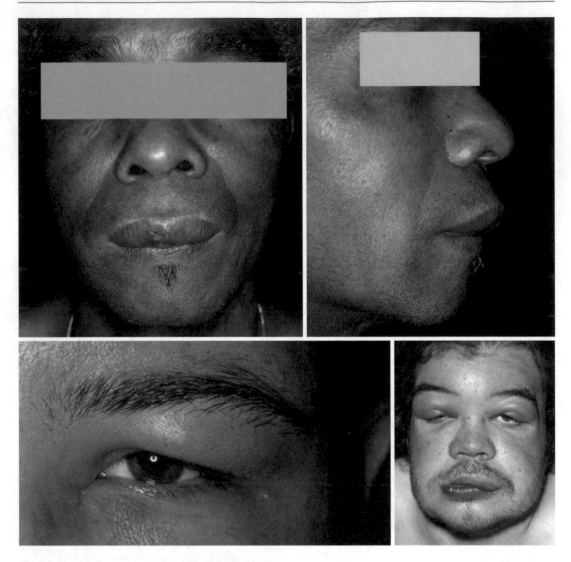

Fig. 10 Angioedema

valsartan, losartan, olmesartan), anti-renin (Alisken).

Alone or associated with:

- **Antidiabetics drugs**: Gliptins (sitagliptin), DDP-IV inhibitors (vildagliptin).
- **Anticancer drugs:** mTOR inhibitors (everolimus, sirolimus).
- **Antipsychotic drugs:** Risperidone.
- **Others**: Vasopeptidase inhibitors (omapatrilat), racecadotril.
• **Lipid-lowering drugs**: Statins: Lovastatin.
• **Hormonal drugs**: Androgens (oral contraceptives, injections, and progesterone implants), anti-hormonal receptor (tamoxifen, raloxifene).
• **Fibrinolytic agents**: Plasminogen activator, streptokinase.

Some drugs may be associated with direct histamine release from mastocyts and basophils; They can induce histaminic angioedema usually associated with urticaria through a direct pharmacologic effect:

- **Nonsteroidal anti-inflammatory drugs (NSAIDs) (+++)**: aspirin (diclofenac, ibuprofen) by altering the metabolism of arachidonic acid.

- **Antimicrobials agents:** B lactamin, vancomycin.
- **Antifungal agents**: Caspofungin.
- **Others**: Opioids or codeine caused by degranulation of mast cells, radiographic contrast media (differential diagnosis: iodide mumps).

10.4 Management

The mainstay in treatment of nonallergic drug-induced angioedema is cessation of the offending agent.

Antihistaminic and corticosteroids can be used for histamine-related angioma but are ineffective in bradykinin-mediated angioedema.

11 Acute Localized Exanthematous Pustulosis

Acute localized exanthematous pustulosis (ALEP) is a localized form of acute generalized exanthematous pustulosis (AGEP). It is a rare variant of acute generalized exanthematous pustulosis (AGEP), also called toxic pustuloderma.

Although, AGEP and ALEP represent an unusually severe cutaneous hypersensitivity reaction to a systemic drug, some cases have also been linked to viral infections, insect bites, plant contact, or airborne allergens.

11.1 Clinical Presentation

It is characterized by acute onset of multiple non-follicular, pinhead-sized, sterile pustules, developed on an erythematous and edematous background, localized typically to face, neck, or chest following drug administration. Skin reaction arises quickly within a few hours, resolving rapidly within a few days without treatment, and it is usually accompanied by fever and neutrophilic leukocytosis (Fig. 11).

11.2 Drug-Induced Acute Localized Exanthematous Pustulosis

- **Antimicrobial drugs**: Penicillin(+++)(amoxicillin +/− clavulanic acid, piperacillin-tazobactam, cefoperazone+/− sulfabactam sodium), macrolides, cephalosporin (Ceftibuten), levofloxacin, trimethoprim-sulfamethoxazole, clindamycin, vancomycin.
- **Antifungal drugs**: Metronidazole.
- **Nonsteroidal anti-inflammatory drugs (NSAIDs) (+++):** Ibuprofen, flurbiprofen, diclofenac.
- **Anticancer drugs:** Docetaxel, sorafenib.
- **Anticonvulsant drugs:** Lamotrigine.
- **Others:** Paracetamol.
- **Hormonal drugs:** Finasteride.
- **Antithrombotic drugs:** Bemiparin.
- **Immunosuppressive drugs:** Infliximab.

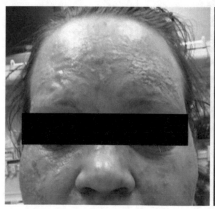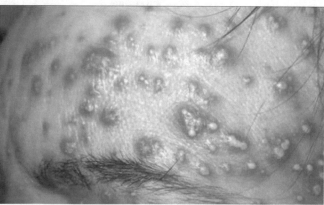

Fig. 11 Acute localized exanthematous pustulosis

11.3   Management

Skin reaction resolves rapidly within a few days without treatment.

Glossary

Drugs	Type of facial adverse events
Anticancer drugs	Bradykinic angioedema, acneiform eruption, SD, Pso, lupus, hirsutism, cheilitis, AELP
5-fluorouracil	Photosensitivity, SD, SCLE, CCLE, rosacea
Adriamycin	SCLE
Bevacizumab	Acneiform eruption
Bortezomib (proteasome inhibitor)	LET
Capecitabine	Photosensitivity
Cetuximab	Hypertrichosis, SD, rosacea, acneiform eruption
Col 3	SCLE
Dabrafenib	SD
Dacarbazine	Photosensitivity
Dasatinib	SD
Docetaxel	SCLE, AELP
Epidermal growth factor receptor inhibitors	Acneiform eruption, rosacea, SD
Epirubicin	Photosensitivity
Erlotinib	Hypertrichosis, rosacea, acneiform eruption, SD
Gefitinib	Hirsutism, SD, acneiform eruption
Hydroxyurea	Photosensitivity
Imatinib	Photosensitivity, Pso, acneiform eruption
Interleukin 2	SD
Ipilimumab	Rosacea
Lapatinib	Rosacea
Leuprorelin	SCLE
Mitomycin	Pso
Nivolumab	Pso, rosacea
Paclitaxel	Photosensitivity, SCLE
Pegylated-liposomal doxorubicin	Pso
Raloxifene	Bradykinic angioedema
Rituximab	Pso
Sorafenib	Pso, SD, cheilitis, acneiform eruption, AELP
Sunitinib	SD

Drugs	Type of facial adverse events
Tyrosine kinase inhibitor	Acneiform eruption
Tamoxifen	Bradykinic angioedema, SCLE
Topical 5-fluorouricil	SD
Trametinib	SD
Vinblastine	Photosensitivity
Vandetanib	Photosensitivity
Vemurafenib	SD, photosensitivity
Anticonvulsants drugs	Pso, SCLE, acneiform eruption, SD, hypertrichosis, AELP
Acetazolamide	Pso
Carbamazepine	Pso, SCLE, acneiform eruption
Lamotrigine	AELP
Levetiracetam	Pso
Phenothiazines	SD, hypertrichosis
Phenytoin	Hypertrichosis, acneiform eruption, SCLE
Sodium valproate	Pso, acneiform eruption
Antidiabetic drugs	Bradykinic angioedema, Pso
DPP-IV inhibitors	Bradykinic angioedema
Glibenclamide	Pso
Gliptins	Bradykinic angioedema
Metformin	Pso
Sitagliptin	Bradykinic angioedema
Vildagliptin	Bradykinic angioedema
Antifungal medications	Histaminic angioedema, photosensitivity, SD, SCLE, Pso, AELP
Caspofungin	Histaminic angioedema
Fluconazole	Photosensitivity
Griseofulvin	SD, photosensitivity, SCLE
Itraconazole	Photosensitivity
Ketoconazole	Photosensibility
Metronidazole	AELP
Terbinafine	SCLE, Pso
Voriconazole	Photosensibility
Antimalarial drugs	Pso, photosensitivity
Chloroquine	Pso
Hydroxychloroquine	Pso
Quinine	Photosensibility
Antimicrobial drugs	Pso, photosensitivity, histaminic angioedema, acneiform eruption, AELP
3rd generation cephalosporins	Photosensitivity
Antituberculosis	Photosensitivity
Amoxicillin+/− Clavulanic acid	AELP

Drugs	Type of facial adverse events
B lactamin	Histaminic angioedema, AELP
Cephalosporin	AELP
Cefoperazone+/− sulfabactam sodium	AELP
Cotrimoxazole	SD
Clindamycin	AELP
Ethionamide	SD
Fluoroquinolones	Photosensitivity, AELP
Hydroxychloroquine	Pso
Isoniazid	Acneiform eruption, photosensibility
Levofloxacin	AELP
Macrolides	Pso, AELP
Penicillin derivated	Pso, AELP
Piperacillin-tazobactam	AELP
Pyrazinamide	Photosensitivity
Sulfonamides derivates	Photosensitivity
Tetracyclines	Photosensitivity, Pso
Trimethoprim-sulfamethoxazole	AELP
Vancomycin	Histaminic angioedema, AELP
Antipsychotics/ neuroleptics drugs	Photosensitivity, acneiform eruption, Pso, SCLE, SD, hypertrichosis
Alprazolam	Photosensitivity
Amineptine	Acneiform eruption
Amitriptyline	Photosensitivity
Aripiprazole	Acneiform eruption
Benzodiazepines	Pso, SCLE
Buspirone	SD
Citalopram	Photosensitivity
Clozapine	Photosensitivity
Clomipramine	Photosensitivity
Chlordiazepoxide	Photosensitivity
Chlorpromazine	SD, photosensitivity
Desipramine	Photosensitivity
Escitalopram	Photosensitivity, acneiform eruption
Fluoxetine	Photosensitivity, Pso
Fluphenazine	Photosensitivity
Fluvoxamine	Photosensitivity
Haloperidol	SD, acneiform eruption
Imipramine	Photosensitivity
Lithium	Acneiform eruption, SD, Pso
Metoclopramide	Hypertrichosis
Olanzapine	Pso, photosensitivity
Paroxetine	Photosensitivity
Perazine	Photosensitivity

Drugs	Type of facial adverse events
Perphenazine	Photosensitivity
Phenelzine	Photosensitivity
Protriptyline	Photosensitivity
Reserpine	Hypertrichosis
Risperidone	Bradykinic angioedema
Sertraline	Photosensitivity, Acneiform eruption
Thiethylperazine	SCLE
Thioridazine	Photosensitivity
Thiothixene	SD
Trazodone	Acneiform eruption
Trifluoperazine	Photosensitivity
Venlafaxine	Pso, photosensitivity
Antithrombotic or fibrinolytic drugs	Bradykinic angioedema, SCLE, AELP
Aspirin	Histaminic angioedema
Bimiparin	AELP
Fibrinolytic agents	Bradykinic angioedema
Plasminogen activator	Bradykinic angioedema
Streptokinase	Bradykinic angioedema
Ticlopidine	SCLE
Antiviral drugs	Photosensitivity, cheilitis, rosacea
Aciclovir (topical)	Photosensitivity)
Efavirenz	Photosensitivity
Indinavir	Cheilitis
Ribavirin	Rosacea
Cardiovascular drugs	SCLE, Pso, LET, rosacea, photosensitivity, bradykinic angioedema, acneiform eruption, hypertrichosis
Aldactone	SCLE
Amiodarone	Pso, photosensitivity
Amlodipine	Photosensitivity
Angiotensin-converting enzyme (ACE) inhibitors	SCLE, Pso, LET, photosensitivity
Anti-renin	Bradykinic angioedema
β-Blockers	Pso, SCLE
Calcium channel blockers	Pso, rosacea, photosensitivity, SCLE
Candesartan	Bradykinic angioedema
Captopril	Bradykinic angioedema, Pso, photosensitivity, SCLE
Chlorthalidone	Pso
Chlorothiazides	SCLE
Cilazapril	SCLE
Cinnarizine	SCLE
Clonidine	Pso
Digoxin	Pso

Drugs	Type of facial adverse events
Diltiazem	Photosensitivity, SCLE
Enalapril	Pso, SCLE, Bradykinic angioedema, photosensitivity
Fibrinolytic agents	Bradykinic angioedema
Furosemide	Photosensitivity
Hydrochlorothiazide +/− triamterene	SCLE, photosensitivity
Indapamide	Photosensitivity
Lisinopril	SCLE, Bradykinic angioedema
Losartan	Bradykinic angioedema
Methyldopa	SD, photosensitivity, hypertrichosis
Nifedipine	Photosensitivity, SCLE
Nitrendipine	SCLE
Olmesartan	Bradykinic angioedema
Omapatrilat	Bradykinic angioedema
Plasminogen activator	Bradykinic angioedema
Quinapril	Photosensitivity
Quinidine	Acneiform eruption, Pso, photosensitivity
Reserpine	Hypertrichosis
Ramipril	Pso, photosensitivity
Rilmenidine	Photosensitivity
Selective phosphodiesterase 5 inhibitors	Rosacea
Streptokinase	Bradykinic angioedema
Tilisolol	Photosensitivity
Thiazide diuretics	Photosensitivity, SCLE
Ticlopidine	SCLE
Triamterene	Photosensitivity
Valsartan	Photosensibility, bradykinic angioedema
Vasopeptidase inhibitors	Bradykinic angioedema
Verapamil	SCLE
H2 antagonist	SD, Pso, SCLE
Cimetidine	SD, Pso
Ranitidine	SCLE
Hormonal drugs	Acneiform eruption, hypertrichosis, SCLE, SD, Pso, AELP
Anabolic steroids	Acneiform eruption, hypertrichosis
Androgens	Acneiform eruption, SD, bradykinic angioedema
Danazol	Acneiform eruption, hypertrichosis
Finasteride	AELP
Leuprorelin	SCLE
Levonorgestrel	Hypertrichosis

Drugs	Type of facial adverse events
Norethindrone	Hypertrichosis
Norgestrel	Hypertrichosis
Progesterone	Acneiform eruption, bradykinic angioedema
Progestins	Hypertrichosis
Raloxifene	Bradykinic angioedema
Tamoxifen	SCLE, bradykinic angioedema
Testosterone	Acneiform eruption, Pso, hypertrichosis
Thyroid medications	SCLE
Immunomodulators drugs	Pso, rosacea, SD, SCLE, hypertrichosis
Imiquimod	Pso
Interferon alpha	Rosacea, SD, Pso, SCLE, hypertrichosis
Interferon beta	Pso, SCLE, hypertrichosis
Immunosuppressive drugs	Acneiform eruption, Pso, CCLE, LET, SCLE, rosacea, hypertrichosis, bradykinic angioedema, AELP
Adalimumab	Pso, SCLE, LET
Azathioprine	Acneiform eruption
Corticosteroids	Acneiform eruption, rosacea, Pso, hypertrichosis
Cyclosporine	Pso, acneiform eruption, hypertrichosis
Efalizumab	SCLE
Etanercept	Rosacea, Pso, SCLE
Everolimus	Bradykinic angioedema
Infliximab	LET, Pso, SCLE, AELP
Lenalidomide	Acneiform eruption
Leflunomide	SCLE
Methotrexate	SCLE
mTOR inhibitors	Bradykinic angioedema, acneiform eruption
Pimecrolimus	Rosacea
Sirolimus	Acneiform eruption, bradykinic angioedema
Tacrolimus	Rosacea
Tumor necrosis factor-alpha inhibitors	Acneiform eruption, Pso, CCLE, LET, SCLE
Lipid-lowering drugs	Bradykinic angioedema, SCLE, photosensitivity, Pso
Atorvastatin	Photosensitivity
Fenofibrates	Photosensitivity, Pso
Gemfibrozil	Psoriasis
Lovastatin	Bradykinic angioedema
Pravastatin	Photosensitivity, SCLE

Drugs	Type of facial adverse events
Simvastatin	Photosensitivity
Statins	Photosensitivity
Nonsteroidal anti-inflammatory drugs	Histaminic angioedema, Pso, SCLE, CCLE, photosensibility, AELP
Aspirin	SCLE, histaminic angioedema
Celecoxib	SCLE
Benzydamine (topical)	Photosensitivity
Diclofenac	Photosensitivity, histaminic angioedema, AELP
Flurbiprofen	AELP
Ibuprofen	Pso, AELP, histaminic angioedema
Indomethacin	Pso
Ketoprofen (topical)	Photosensitivity
Meclofenamate	Pso
Naproxen	SCLE, Pso
Piroxicam	Photosensitivity, SCLE
Phenylbutazone	Pso
Others	–
Botulinum A toxin	Pso
Bupropion	SCLE
Codeine	Histaminic angioedema
Fluoride dentifrice	POD
Gold	SD
Halogens	Photosensitivity, acneiform eruption
Heroin	Cheilitis
Icodextrin	Pso
Iodine	Hypertrichosis
Methamphetamine	Cheilitis
Methoxsalen	SD
Minoxidil	Hypertrichosis
Opioids	Histaminic angioedema
Oral parabens	Rosacea
Paracetamol	AELP
Psoralens	SD
Pyridoxine	Rosacea, acneiform eruption
Racecadotril	Bradykinic angioedema
Radiographic contrast media	Histaminic angioedema
Recombinant granulocyte-macrophage colony stimulating factors	Psoriasis
Tiotropium	SCLE
Vitamin B complex	Rosacea, acneiform eruption
Prostaglandin analogue	Hirsutism

Drugs	Type of facial adverse events
Bimatoprost	Hirsutism
Latanoprost	Hirsutism
Proton pump inhibitor	SCLE
Lansoprazole	SCLE
Omeprazole	SCLE
Pantoprazole	CCLE
Vitamin A derivative	Cheilitis
Isotretinoin	SD

AELP acute localized exanthematous pustulosis, *CCLE* chronic cutaneous lupus erythematosus, *LET* lupus erythematosus tumidus, *POD* perioral dermatitis, *Pso* psoriasis, *SCLE* subacute cutaneous lupus erythematous, *SD* seborrheic dermatitis

Bibliography

Arrizabalaga M, Casanueva T, Benítez J, Escribano G, Gallardo C. Massive secondary psoriasiform dermatitis secondary to intravesical administration of mitomycin C. Arch Esp Urol. 1989;42(7):670–2.

Barzilai A, David M, Trau H, Hodak E. Seborrheic dermatitis-like eruption in patients taking isotretinoin therapy for acne: retrospective study of five patients. Am J Clin Dermatol. 2008;9(4):255–61.

Benomar S, Boutayeb S, Afifi Y, Hamada S, Bouhllab J, Hassam B, et al. Hand-foot syndrome and seborrheic dermatitis-like eruption induced by erlotinib. Dermatol Online J. 2009;15(11):2.

Berk T, Scheinfeld N. Seborrheic dermatitis. Pharm Ther. 2010;35(6):348–52.

Bettoli V, Mantovani L, Boccia S, Virgili A. Rosacea fulminans related to pegylated interferon alpha-2b and ribavirin therapy. Acta Derm Venereol. 2006;86(3):258–9.

Binder RL, Jonelis FJ. Seborrheic dermatitis: a newly reported side effect of neuroleptics. J Clin Psychiatry. 1984;45(3):125–6.

Bousquet E, Zarbo A, Tournier E, Chevreau C, Mazieres J, Lacouture ME, et al. Development of Papulopustular rosacea during Nivolumab therapy for metastatic cancer. Acta Derm Venereol. 2017;97(4):539–40.

Bowden JB, Rapini RP. Psoriasiform eruption from intramuscular botulinum A toxin. Cutis. 1992;50(6):415–6.

Brenner S, Cabili S, Wolf R. Widespread erythematous scaly plaques in an adult. Psoriasiform eruption induced by quinidine. Arch Dermatol. 1993;129(10):1331–2, 1334-5

Brenner S, Golan H, Lerman Y. Psoriasiform eruption and anticonvulsant drugs. Acta Derm Venereol. 2000;80(5):382.

Brodell EE, Smith E, Brodell RT. Exacerbation of seborrheic dermatitis by topical fluorouracil. Arch Dermatol. 2011;147(2):245–6.

Chen H-M. Patients' experiences and perceptions of chemotherapy-induced oral mucositis in a day unit. Cancer Nurs. 2008;31(5):363–9.

Chepure AH, Ungratwar AK. Olanzapine-induced psoriasis. Indian J Psychol Med. 2017;39(6):811–2.

Cho SG, Park YM, Moon H, Kim KM, Bae SS, Kim GB, et al. Psoriasiform eruption triggered by recombinant granulocyte-macrophage colony stimulating factor (rGM-CSF) and exacerbated by granulocyte colony stimulating factor (rG-CSF) in a patient with breast cancer. J Korean Med Sci. 1998;13(6):685–8.

Cohen AD, Bonneh DY, Reuveni H, Vardy DA, Naggan L, Halevy S. Drug exposure and psoriasis vulgaris: case-control and case-crossover studies. Acta Derm Venereol. 2005;85(4):299–303.

Cuétara MS, Aguilar A, Martin L, Aspiroz C, del Palacio A. Erlotinib associated with rosacea-like folliculitis and Malassezia sympodialis. Br J Dermatol. 2006;155(2):477–9.

Dalle S, Becuwe C, Balme B, Thomas L. Venlafaxine-associated psoriasiform palmoplantar keratoderma and subungual hyperkeratosis. Br J Dermatol. 2006;154(5):999–1000.

David M, Livni E, Stern E, Feuerman EJ, Grinblatt J. Psoriasiform eruption induced by digoxin: confirmed by re-exposure. J Am Acad Dermatol. 1981;5(6):702–3.

Dika E, Ravaioli GM, Fanti PA, Piraccini BM, Lambertini M, Chessa MA, et al. Cutaneous adverse effects during ipilimumab treatment for metastatic melanoma: a prospective study. Eur J Dermatol. 2017;27(3):266–70.

Fry L, Baker BS. Triggering psoriasis: the role of infections and medications. Clin Dermatol. 2007;25(6):606–15.

Gencler OS, Gencler B, Altunel CT, Arslan N. Levetiracetam induced psoriasiform drug eruption: a rare case report. Saudi Pharm J SPJ Off Publ Saudi Pharm Soc. 2015;23(6):720–2.

Gerber PA, Kukova G, Buhren BA, Homey B. Density of Demodex folliculorum in patients receiving epidermal growth factor receptor inhibitors. Dermatology. 2011;222(2):144–7.

Giard C, Nicolie B, Drouet M, Lefebvre-Lacoeuille C, Le Sellin J, Bonneau J-C, et al. Angio-oedema induced by oestrogen contraceptives is mediated by bradykinin and is frequently associated with urticaria. Dermatology. 2012;225(1):62–9.

Goh CL. Psoriasiform drug eruption due to glibenclamide. Australas J Dermatol. 1987;28(1):30–2.

Gómez Torrijos E, Cortina de la Calle MP, Méndez Díaz Y, Moreno Lozano L, Extremera Ortega A, Galindo Bonilla PA, et al. Acute Localized Exanthematous Pustulosis Due to Bemiparin. J Investig Allergol Clin Immunol. 2017;27(5):328–9.

Graves JE, Jones BF, Lind AC, Heffernan MP. Nonscarring inflammatory alopecia associated with the epidermal growth factor receptor inhibitor gefitinib. J Am Acad Dermatol. 2006;55(2):349–53.

Haddock ES, Cohen PR. 5-Fluorouracil-induced exacerbation of rosacea. Dermatol Online J. 2016; 22(11).

Henningsen E, Bygum A. Budesonide-induced periorificial dermatitis presenting as chalazion and blepharitis. Pediatr Dermatol. 2011;28(5):596–7.

Hopkins Z, Frigerio A, Clarke JT. Acute localized exanthematous pustulosis (ALEP) caused by lamotrigine. JAAD Case Rep. 2018;4(7):645–7.

Ioannides D, Lazaridou E, Apalla Z, Devliotou-Panagiotidou D. Phosphodiesterase-5 inhibitors and rosacea: report of 10 cases. Br J Dermatol. 2009;160(3):719–20.

Jansen T, Romiti R, Kreuter A, Altmeyer P. Rosacea fulminans triggered by high-dose vitamins B6 and B12. J Eur Acad Dermatol Venereol. 2001;15(5):484–5.

Kanwar AJ, Majid A, Garg MP, Singh G. Seborrheic dermatitis-like eruption caused by cimetidine. Arch Dermatol. 1981;117(2):65–6.

Katz M, Seidenbaum M, Weinrauch L. Penicillin-induced generalized pustular psoriasis. J Am Acad Dermatol. 1987;17(5 Pt 2):918–20.

Kawakami Y, Nakamura-Wakatsuki T, Yamamoto T. Seborrheic dermatitis-like eruption following interleukin-2 administration. Dermatol Online J. 2010;16(9):12.

Kazandjieva J, Tsankov N. Drug-induced acne. Clin Dermatol. 2017;35(2):156–62.

Kim GK, Del Rosso JQ. Drug-provoked psoriasis: is it drug induced or drug aggravated?: understanding pathophysiology and clinical relevance. J Clin Aesthetic Dermatol. 2010;3(1):32–8.

Koca R, Altinyazar HC, Yenidünya S, Tekin NS. Psoriasiform drug eruption associated with metformin hydrochloride: a case report. Dermatol Online J. 2003;9(3):11.

Köstler WJ, Hejna M, Wenzel C, Zielinski CC. Oral mucositis complicating chemotherapy and/or radiotherapy: options for prevention and treatment. CA Cancer J Clin. 2001;51(5):290–315.

Kreuter A, Gambichler T, Schlottmann R, Altmeyer P, Brockmeyer N. Psoriasiform pustular eruptions from pegylated-liposomal doxorubicin in AIDS-related Kaposi's sarcoma. Acta Derm Venereol. 2001;81(3):224.

Lambert D, Beer F, Gisselman R, Bouilly D, Chapuis JL. Cutaneous lesions due to lithium therapy (author's transl). Ann Dermatol Venereol. 1982;109(1):19–24.

Laurinaviciene R, Sandholdt LH, Bygum A. Drug-induced cutaneous lupus erythematosus: 88 new cases. Eur J Dermatol. 2017;27(1):28–33.

Lerch M, Mainetti C, Terziroli Beretta-Piccoli B, Harr T. Current perspectives on Stevens-Johnson syndrome and toxic epidermal necrolysis. Clin Rev Allergy Immunol. 2018;54(1):147–76.

Lipozenčić J, Hadžavdić SL. Perioral dermatitis. Clin Dermatol. 2014;32(1):125–30.

Martín JM, Pellicer Z, Bella R, Jordá E. Rosacea triggered by a vitamin B complex supplement. Actas Dermosifiliogr. 2011;102(3):223–4.

Michaelis TC, Sontheimer RD, Lowe GC. An update in drug-induced subacute cutaneous lupus erythematosus. Dermatol Online J. 2017;23(3).

Mokos ZB, Kummer A, Mosler EL, Čeović R, Basta-Juzbašić A. Perioral dermatitis: still a therapeutic challenge. Acta Clin Croat. 2015;54(2):179–85.

Momin SB, Peterson A, Del Rosso JQ. A status report on drug-associated acne and acneiform eruptions. J Drugs Dermatol. 2010;9(6):627–36.

Monteiro AF, Rato M, Martins C. Drug-induced photosensitivity: Photoallergic and phototoxic reactions. Clin Dermatol. 2016;34(5):571–81.

Ocvirk J, Heeger S, McCloud P, Hofheinz R-D. A review of the treatment options for skin rash induced by EGFR-targeted therapies: evidence from randomized clinical trials and a meta-analysis. Radiol Oncol. 2013;47(2):166–75.

Peralta L, Morais P. Perioral dermatitis—the role of nasal steroids. Cutan Ocul Toxicol. 2012;31(2): 160–3.

Peters P, Drummond C. Perioral dermatitis from high fluoride dentifrice: a case report and review of literature. Aust Dent J. 2013;58(3):371–2.

Rezaković S, Bukvić Mokos Z, Paštar Z. Drug-induced rosacea-like dermatitis. Acta Dermatovenerol Croat. 2016a;24(1):49–54.

Rezaković S, Mokos ZB, Paštar Z. Pyridoxine induced rosacea-like dermatitis. Acta Clin Croat. 2015;54(1):99–102.

Rezaković S, Paštar Z, Bukvić Mokos Z, Pavliša G, Kovačević S. Erlotinib-induced rosacea-like dermatitis. Acta Dermatovenerol Croat. 2016b;24(1):65–9.

Riahi RR, Cohen PR. Dasatinib-induced Seborrheic dermatitis-like eruption. J Clin Aesthetic Dermatol. 2017;10(7):23–7.

Sehgal VN, Dogra S, Srivastava G, Aggarwal AK. Psoriasiform dermatoses. Indian J Dermatol Venereol Leprol. 2008;74(2):94–9.

Senilă S, Seicean A, Fechete O, Grad A, Ungureanu L. Infliximab-induced acne and acute localized exanthematous pustulosis: case report. Dermatol Ther. 2017;30(6).

Stone C, Brown NJ. Angiotensin-converting enzyme inhibitor and other drug-associated angioedema. Immunol Allergy Clin North Am. 2017;37(3):483–95.

Techasatian L, Panombualert S, Uppala R, Jetsrisuparb C. Drug-induced Stevens-Johnson syndrome and toxic epidermal necrolysis in children: 20 years study in a tertiary care hospital. World J Pediatr. 2017;13(3):255–60.

Troyanova-Slavkova S, Eickenscheidt L, Dumann K, Kowalzick L. Initially undetected de novo psoriasis triggered by nivolumab for metastatic base of the tongue carcinoma. Hautarzt. 2018;69(8):674–80.

Tsankov N, Botev-Zlatkov N, Lazarova AZ, Kostova M, Popova L, Tonev S. Psoriasis and drugs: influence of tetracyclines on the course of psoriasis. J Am Acad Dermatol. 1988;19(4):629–32.

Valance A, Lebrun-Vignes B, Descamps V, Queffeulou G, Crickx B. Icodextrin cutaneous hypersensitivity: report of 3 psoriasiform cases. Arch Dermatol. 2001;137(3):309–10.

Villani A, Baldo A, De Fata Salvatores G, Desiato V, Ayala F, Donadio C. Acute localized Exanthematous Pustulosis (ALEP): review of literature with report of case caused by amoxicillin-Clavulanic acid. Dermatol Ther. 2017;7(4):563–70.

Wehrmann C, Sondermann W, Körber A. Secukinumab-induced subacute-cutaneous lupus erythematosus. Hautarzt. 2018;69(1):64–6.

Wolf R, Dorfman B, Krakowski A. Psoriasiform eruption induced by captopril and chlorthalidone. Cutis. 1987;40(2):162–4.

Yang C-H, Lin W-C, Chuang C-K, Chang Y-C, Pang S-T, Lin Y-C, et al. Hand-foot skin reaction in patients treated with sorafenib: a clinicopathological study of cutaneous manifestations due to multitargeted kinase inhibitor therapy. Br J Dermatol. 2008;158(3): 592–6.

Yazici A, Akturk AS, Cefle A, Bayramgurler D, Yildiz KD. Rosacea associated with etanercept. Joint Bone Spine Rev Rhum. 2014;81(3):274–5.

Conclusion: Drug-Induced Oral Complications

Sarah Cousty and Sara Laurencin-Dalicieux

As previously stated, adverse drug reactions (ADR) are unwanted, undesirable, sometimes unpredictable effects that can occur during the clinical use of medication. No drug can be considered totally exempt of potential side effects. These effects can manifest themselves either on the first intake of the drug or after continuous usage even in standard forms of dosage and may develop by a direct or indirect physiological mechanism. The prevalence increases with age especially due to polymedication related to the multiple pathologies of the elderly.

The oral manifestations linked to the most commonly prescribed drugs have been presented and described in the different chapters of this book.

The mouth, like the skin, can be one of the first indicators of changes due to medication. However, these manifestations are often underdiagnosed, underestimated, and misjudged which

lead to delayed diagnoses and can have a major impact on patients' quality of life and well-being. Several reasons could explain this:

- The lack of reports to the pharmacovigilance centers.
- Inaccurate lesion description or the use of nonspecific terminologies such as "stomatitis," "mucositis," "aphthous ulcerations," "mucosal inflammation."

Some medications have a greater ability to cause adverse oral reactions. Xerostomia, taste disturbances, and ulceration are among the numerous specific adverse drug complications. Unfortunately, most of the time, reactions are nonspecific as they can mimic particular oral diseases such as bullous diseases (including autoimmune mucous epithelial or subepithelial diseases such as pemphigus or pemphigoid) or oral lichen planus. Adverse drug reactions may affect the oral mucosa or the alveolar bone. More recent reports point out the risk of osteonecrosis of the jaw with the use of bisphosphonates, or lichenoid mucosal lesions with the use of targeted therapies, for example. For the dentist, gingival overgrowth is the most well-known adverse oral complication.

When confronted with a patient complaining of stomatitis, ulceration and necrosis, opportunistic infections, hemorrhage, gingival hyperplasia, pigmentation, altered salivary function, or altered taste sensation, reviewing his medical record regarding his medication is essential. Drug

S. Cousty (✉)
Oral Surgery Oral Medecine Department, Dental Faculty, Paul Sabatier University, Toulouse, France

Oral Surgery Oral Medecine Department, CHU de Toulouse, Toulouse, France

LAPLACE, UMR CNRS 5213, Paul Sabatier University, Toulouse, France

S. Laurencin-Dalicieux
Periodontology Department, Dental Faculty, Paul Sabatier University, Toulouse, France

Periodontology Department, CHU de Toulouse, Toulouse, France

CERPOP, UMR INSERM 1295, Paul Sabatier University, Toulouse, France removal or substitution is the best and safest way to resolve the clinical problem.

Unfortunately, this is not always possible and some drugs cannot be substituted, especially in the field of oncology. For these reasons, as continuously new molecules become part of the therapeutic arsenal, prescription in the field of oncology is very particular, and management protocols are frequently updated and adjusted to compensate and try to limit the complications associated with the molecules or procedures. Conventional cancer chemotherapies induce various and multiple oral side effects such as mucositis, hyposalivation/xerostomia, dysphagia, taste alteration, ulcerations, or infections. As far as cancer management and adverse drug reactions are considered, targeted cancer therapies represent a real therapeutic progress. They are generally much better tolerated by patients and do not induce the "classical"—quality of life impairing—adverse effects usually observed with cytotoxic chemotherapy.

However, they can still present some oral cavity complications. The main ones are mentioned in the following table.

M-TORR inhibitor	Stomatitis, ulcerations
EGFR/HER inhibitor	Stomatitis, ulcerations
MEK inhibitor	Stomatitis, ulcerations
Tyrosine kinase inhibitor	Stomatitis, ulcerations, benign migratory glossitis, mucosal pigmentation, osteonecrosis of the jaw
BRAF inhibitor	Hyperkeratotic lesions
BCR ABL inhibitors	Lichenoid lesions, mucosal pigmentation
Anti-CD20	Lichenoid lesions
Immune checkpoint inhibitors (anti PD-1, anti PDL-1)	Lichenoid lesions
Anti-VEGF	Benign migratory glossitis

Another future challenge, in the field of drug-induced oral complications, is the management of the elderly and polymedicated patients. Adverse drug reactions are, on average, twice as common in the older individual than in younger adults. Ageing is accompanied by an increase in the prevalence of diseases (cardiometabolic, neurological, osteoarticular, respiratory, ocular, renal, etc.) that are often associated with or a complication of each other. Hence administration of several specific drugs is frequent, the consequences of which are often more serious (hospitalization, death), and highlighting the drug responsible is more difficult. Also the elderly patient is also more sensitive to adverse drug reactions as these effects relate to cellular aging (skin, eye, central nervous system, etc.) or altered organ functions (liver, kidney). In the elderly, cardiovascular drugs are the most frequently involved in adverse reactions. One of the reasons why is that they are the most prescribed.

This book presents an overview of different drug-induced oral complications. The lesions induced by these drugs can significantly alter the patient's oral function, comfort, and quality of life.

Many oral drug effects are well documented and even reported by manufacturers on the drug's explanatory note. However, new medications (such as targeted therapies) continuously marketed and the increase in polymedicated patients, especially in the elderly, made it difficult to be exhaustive. Pharmacology resources are available to support decision-making in particular in the evaluation of risk management. Practitioners (oral specialists, dentists, and others) should also be aware of differential diagnosis of oral mucosa lesions and beware of confounding clinical pictures while always taking into consideration patients' complaints. Even if drug treatment interruption or replacement can be complicated, it should be discussed with the prescribing practitioner with regard to the patient's benefit/risk ratio. Additional research is needed to support and develop better practices and guidelines to minimize and manage the oral consequences of medication use.

Bibliography

Molina-Guarneros JA, Sainz-Gil M, Sanz Fadrique R, García P, Rodríguez-Jiménez P, Navarro-García E, Martin LH. Bullous pemphigoid associated with the use of dipeptidil peptidase-4 inhibitors: analysis from studies based on pharmacovigilance databases. Int J Clin Pharm. 2020;42(2):713–20. https://doi.org/10.1007/s11096-020-01003-6.

Shah N, Cohen L, Seminario-Vidal L. Management of oral reactions from immune checkpoint inhibitor therapy: a systematic review. J Am Acad Dermatol. 2020;83(5):1493–8. https://doi.org/10.1016/j.jaad.2020.05.133.

Watters AL, et al. Oral complications of targeted cancer therapies: a narrative literature review. Oral Oncol. 2011;47(6):441–8.

Index

© Springer Nature Switzerland AG 2021
S. Cousty, S. Laurencin-Dalicieux (eds.), *Drug-Induced Oral Complications*,
https://doi.org/10.1007/978-3-030-66973-7

Printed in the United States
by Baker & Taylor Publisher Services